I0039329

THE WELLNESS DIABETES COACH

11 Secrets to Improve Your Health in 90 Days

PAULINE M. BRYAN

10-10-10
Publishing

The Wellness Diabetes Coach: 11 Secrets to Improve Your Health in 90 Days

www.wellnesscoachbook.com

Copyright © 2021 Pauline M. Bryan

ISBN: 978-1-77277-409-2

All rights reserved. No portion of this book may be reproduced mechanically, electronically, or by any other means, including photocopying, without permission of the publisher or author except in the case of brief quotations embodied in critical articles and reviews. It is illegal to copy this book, post it to a website, or distribute it by any other means without permission from the publisher or author.

References to internet websites (URLs) were accurate at the time of writing. Authors and the publishers are not responsible for URLs that may have expired or changed since the manuscript was prepared.

Limits of Liability and Disclaimer of Warranty

The author and publisher shall not be liable for your misuse of the enclosed material. This book is strictly for informational and educational purposes only.

Warning – Disclaimer

The purpose of this book is to educate and entertain. The author and/or publisher do not guarantee that anyone following these techniques, suggestions, tips, ideas, or strategies will become successful. The author and/or publisher shall have neither liability nor responsibility to anyone with respect to any loss or damage caused, or alleged to be caused, directly or indirectly by the information contained in this book.

Medical Disclaimer

The medical or health information in this book is provided as an information resource only, and is not to be used or relied on for any diagnostic or treatment purposes. This information is not intended to be patient education, does not create any patient-physician relationship, and should not be used as a substitute for professional diagnosis and treatment.

Publisher
10-10-10 Publishing
Markham, ON
Canada

Printed in Canada and the United States of America

DEDICATION

I dedicate this book to my beautiful and loving sister, Dona Marilyn Mason. I am lucky to have been given the gift of having you in my life to walk beside me. I miss you every day.

TABLE OF CONTENTS

FOREWORD

Have you been diagnosed with diabetes? Are you feeling overwhelmed with all of the information out there? Do you want to feel better but you're not sure where to start? Are you ready to take your life back, and take control of your health?

No matter where you are in your journey to better health and living a more fulfilling life every single day, *The Wellness Diabetes Coach* is filled with insights that will guide you every step of the way. As you read each chapter you will gain knowledge that will make it easier for you to progress to the next step. This book is a complete guide to getting your health back on track.

Author Pauline Bryan makes it easy for you to achieve the healthy lifestyle you desire by providing easy to follow tips and tricks. She lives by example. Her lifelong mission to live a life of optimal health has led her to create a program that makes sense for your everyday life.

Her experience, helping her sister navigate her life and journey to better health after a diabetes diagnosis, has inspired her to share her knowledge with you. She takes your desire to make your health a priority, and makes it a reality. Better health does get to be easy, especially when you give yourself the tools you need to succeed. This book is one of the best.

Pauline generously shares some of her favorite recipes to help you learn how to make delicious healthy options. She believes that when you enjoy the food you are eating it is easier to make a choice to eat in a way that helps your body thrive. You will learn how to change your perspective on what you eat, and how to provide yourself with snacks that are good for you.

You will also find useful tips to help you manage your medication, get more social, keep your personal hygiene in check so that you feel great about yourself, and get more active. Pauline's approach is all about fun. When you make your healthy lifestyle fun to achieve, then you are sure to succeed.

Get ready to wake up, each and every day, feeling alive and ready for life!

Raymond Aaron
New York Times Bestselling Author

CHAPTER 1

Healthy Body, Healthy Mind, Healthy Life

Everything Starts with Health

"Everyone has their own definition of a healthy lifestyle, and mine has come to mean making health a priority but not an obsession."

– Daphne Oz

1

Value Your Life

You may be here for a long time.
You may be here for a short time.
Your life is yours.

And while there are many things you will not have control over, you will always have control over your response to those things. You will always have control over how you choose to live each day. You will always have control over how much you value your own life.

I believe that if you learn to value your life in the very moment you are living, regardless of the hurdles you have overcome, you will ultimately realize that you need to be kind to your body. If you truly value each day you are here, you know that your health matters. The better you are to your body, the more you are able to enjoy the moment without chronic pain or illness.

I know I am not telling you anything new. Also, I know you may be wondering what all of this has to do with maintaining your diabetes. It is simple: If you learn how to value your life, you will begin to understand that you are the one and only person who can get your health under control.

A healthy lifestyle begins with you. That being said, you can always look outside yourself for support, guidance, and knowledge. You have to be the one to take control, but that does not ever mean you have to do it alone. This book will help you understand what kind of help you need, find the help you need, and learn how to ask for it. Getting support on your journey to becoming a healthier version of yourself will, without a doubt, help ensure greater success and a whole lot more fun along the way.

It is Time to Thrive

You picked up this book because you are ready to take control of your life. You know that you could be doing much better. You understand that it is time for you to take action. Ultimately, you are reading this book because you want to live the best life you can.

Life is not simply about getting by from day to day. You have a lot of living to do, and you can not do that when you are exhausted and worried all the time. Living in the moment means doing the very best you can to feel great about yourself, your choices, and your daily activities. Sure, there will always be things we can not control, but choosing a healthier lifestyle is on you!

A lot of the literature on diabetes that is available talks about managing your condition. I do not agree with this at all. I do not want you to simply manage. I do not want you to simply get by. Life is not just about surviving.

I WANT YOU TO THRIVE!

You can thrive! Even with diabetes, you can thrive!

My 11-step program is to establish a healthier lifestyle after diabetes, which involves a lot more than just eating right. But all of it is simple and achievable. In this book, I will share some of the ways in which I help my clients achieve greater health within 90 days, by addressing the following:

1. Diet

What are your current eating habits?

How are they negatively affecting your diabetes symptoms?

What can you do to change your eating habits to achieve better health?

2. Exercise

How active are you in your daily life?

What physical activities do you enjoy doing?

3. Hygiene

What is your daily hygiene routine?

How can hygiene affect the way you feel about yourself?

Why does hygiene matter?

4. Monitoring

Are you aware of your habits?

How do you monitor your health?

How can you start monitoring yourself more effectively?

5. Socialize

Why does being social matter to your overall health?

How social are you?

What social activities do you love?

6. Family Support

Do you have the support you need to live a healthier lifestyle?

Do you know what kind of support you need?

Do you know how to ask for support?

In order to shift from your current habits to new, healthier habits, there is one thing you need to do: shift your mindset! It is simple, but it takes work. You will notice there is a theme to my overall message: it is simple, but it takes work! One of the best things you can do for yourself is to stop thinking that adopting new healthy habits is hard. It does not have to be. It can be easy. It is all up to you.

Set Your Mind Straight

> *"Open the window of your mind. Allow the fresh air, new lights, and new truths to enter."*

> **– Amit Ray**

Changing your lifestyle is a challenge; but again, it does not have to be hard. You truly can do anything you set your mind to. But you have to commit to setting your mind to it. What does this mean exactly?

It means you have to be willing to change. It is simple, but it takes work. Setting your mind to living a healthy lifestyle happens in three easy steps:

1. Recognize your desire for change.

2. Understand the thought patterns that are keeping you stuck.

3. Change your thought patterns to reflect the change that you want.

Have you ever thought of something you wanted to do to positively change your life in some way, and then promptly went on to keep doing the thing you always do, which goes against the positive change you just wanted to make. It is easy to think we want to do something, but in order to actually follow through with it, we need to recognize why we desire the change, and how strong our desire is for the change.

If your desire comes in the form of an easily discarded, passing thought, you most likely will not follow through. So if you find yourself wanting to make a change for the better, take some time and explore that desire. Sit down and write about the desired change.

Here are a few writing prompts to get you going:

1. What is my desire? Define it clearly.

2. How long have I had this desire?

3. Why do I have this desire?

4. If I were to successfully realize this desire, how would it positively change my life?

5. How much do I want this change in my life?

Here is an example to help you out:

What is my desire?

I want to eat healthier.

How long have I had this desire?

It has been with me longer than I can remember. I started gaining a significant amount of weight in my late 40s, and when it first started happening, I thought that it was normal for someone my age to gain weight, but it was bothering me. I was eating the way that I always did, but my body seemed to be processing it differently. I did not want to change the way I ate. Food is a comfort for me and, at the time, I did not want to lose that comfort. It has been such a slow, long build that changing it feels overwhelming. I worry that I have let it go too far.

Why do I have this desire?

I want to feel better. I feel like I am missing out on so many good things in life because I am tired all the time. I get out of breath climbing a few short stairs, and have a hard time playing with my grandchildren. I feel so uncomfortable in both my body and my clothes. I hate feeling this way. I want to feel good about myself and the way I look.

If I were to successfully realize this desire, how would it positively change my life?

I would feel better.

I had to stop saying no to fancy events because I do not have anything to wear.

I had to be able to run around the backyard with my grandchildren.

I had felt less worried about my health.

I would know that I did my best to be here for my family.

I would feel a sense of pride in my accomplishments.

How much do I want this change in my life?

I have been wanting this for so long. I cannot stop thinking about it. It is more than a want; it is a desire. I am ready to do the work. I am ready to feel great about myself and my health.

Next, you need to understand some of the thought patterns that are keeping you stuck, and change those thought patterns to reflect the change that you want to make in your life. These are both larger topics that we will delve into later in the book. For now, I want you to pull out your journal at least once a day and write out your desire, no less than ten times. As you write, feel that desire radiate from the top of your head to the tips of your toes. This will be the affirmation you work with over the course of this book.

Throughout the day, you should say this desire to yourself as often as you remember. If you find yourself forgetting, why not set a timer on your phone to remind you. Set it for at least five times a day.

Ditch the All or Nothing Thinking

No one is perfect, and neither are you! When people fall back into their old behavioral patterns, they give up because they feel like they have failed.

If you love sugary drinks, and you succeeded in not drinking them for three days straight, but you succumb to the craving for one on the fourth day, it does not mean you failed. Let me repeat that: If you fall off the wagon once, it does not mean that you have failed.

You can always get back on the wagon. It is never too late to live a healthy life. And it does not have to be hard. You just have to have a strong and unwavering desire. Remember your desire. Speak it out loud. Do not lose sight of it, and never let it go.

Find the Support You Need

"Be strong, be fearless, be beautiful. And believe that anything is possible when you have the right people there to support you."

– Misty Copeland

One of the best things you can do for yourself is to find the support you need. As you embark on your journey to a healthier lifestyle, you will find yourself facing many challenges. These will come in many different forms:

- Negative self-talk

- Low confidence levels

- Unexpected life circumstances

- Lack of acceptance from friends and loved ones

These are just to name a few. One of the best ways you can arm yourself to take on these challenges is to find a team of supporters who will have your back every step of the way. This book will help you find your support network and learn how to ask for help.

As much as our family and friends love us, and often feel that they have our best interests at heart, sometimes that is not always the case. People are resistant to change. It is normal. They love you for who you are, and as much as they want you to be happy, they may be resistant to you not fitting in the nice neat box they have placed you in. Also, for some, they could see your positive changes as a threat to their own lifestyle. I will share some of my tips for understanding who in your network you can depend on for support, and how to ask for the support you need.

I will also share some knowledge on how to find outside support when you need it, as well as how to deflect some of the negative feedback you may face as you change your health for the better.

Be the Support

"There is no exercise better for the heart than reaching down and lifting people up."

– John Holmes

This book is not only for those who have been diagnosed with diabetes. It is also for those who want to support family or friends along on their journey to achieving a healthier lifestyle. If someone you love needs your help, guidance, or inspiration, there are so many ways that you can be there for them. Here are a few to get you started:

1. **Lead by example** – The best way to help those closest to you get healthier, is to get healthier yourself. I can help. In reading this book, you

will gain more knowledge on how you, too, can lead a healthier life.

2. **Remove all obstacles** – If they need you to remove all sugary drinks from the house in the beginning, do that for them. If you are not ready to give them up, you can always have the sugary drink away from them, outside your home.

3. **Listen** – Hear them out. Changing your life can bring up a lot of emotions. They may need a soft shoulder or a kind ear to depend on as they work through some of the things that come up.

4. **Have fun together** – This one is easy. Make the time to do things you enjoy together.

You have the opportunity to be someone's light. If you choose to take it, you could be the one thing that gets your loved one through a dark day.

My Sister, My Inspiration

"A sister is worth a thousand friends."

– **Unknown**

My sister's love of life was one of the most inspiring things about her. No matter how many struggles she faced, or how she could have let this world bring her down, she did not. She was a free-spirited girl in a woman's body, who loved her family to the moon and back. Although sometimes shy, she loved people and had a lot of friends.

One of my favorite memories was when we were getting ready to go out on the town one night. She lived a good plane ride away, so this was during one of her visits, which always made me happy. Just as we were about to leave, I looked at her and smiled. "Do you think you should iron the wrinkles out of that shirt?"

"Oh no, I do not need to do that; my body will iron them for me!"

We looked at each other and laughed and laughed. She was and still is an incredibly beautiful soul.

I miss her every single day, and I am so incredibly grateful that out of all the sisters she could have had on this vast planet, she was mine. She always looked up to me and followed my guidance. It felt good. I knew that I was able to have a positive impact on her life.

Later in her life, she was diagnosed with diabetes. She was not managing her health well, which only served to make her symptoms worse. I worried and wished she had the support at home to make her health a priority. When she was with me, things were different. I stopped her from drinking pop (soda, if you are in the US), and fed her healthy meals rather than the fast food she often chose.

We also had fun and laughed. We lived. This is such a huge component to living a healthy life, and it is one that can often be overlooked. Thriving after a diabetes diagnosis is not just about getting exercise and eating well; it is also about living well.

The idea of living well means different things to everyone. I am not here to tell you how to live. I am here to inspire you to live your healthiest life in all ways: physical, emotional, spiritual, and… well, I do not know how to say this other than to ask—how does your life measure up on the fun scale? You need to take some time to have fun. Do the things you love! Get out there and dance in the rain. Get up at dawn and watch the sun rise over the horizon. Go to the movies. Do what makes you happy.

That is what my sister inspired me to do, and that is why I am writing this book. I have always placed huge importance on living a healthy lifestyle. Do not get me wrong; I fell off the wagon sometimes. I am not perfect. But I have overcome my fair share of illness, and I am here to share with you how I did it. I eat real food. I do not want a lot of bad sugars. I laugh. I accept support. I seek help when I need it. I share my knowledge with others. Stick with me, and you will have a better idea of what a healthy lifestyle looks like for you.

Just in Case You Didn't Know

Let's take a brief moment to look at some of the statistics the World Health Organization has shared on diabetes globally. Do not worry, this is the last time we will do this! It is good for you to know but not good for you to dwell on. I see this kind of information as a motivator. It is a motivator for you to not be a number. You are not your diabetes!

So, here are a few facts based on research published by the World Health Organization in October 2018:

- The number of people with diabetes has risen from 108 million in 1980, to 422 million in 2014.

- The global prevalence of diabetes* among adults over 18 years of age has risen from 4.7% in 1980, to 8.5% in 2014 (1).

- Diabetes prevalence has been rising more rapidly in middle and low-income countries.

- Diabetes is a major cause of blindness, kidney failure, heart attacks, stroke, and lower limb amputation.

- In 2016, an estimated 1.6 million deaths were directly caused by diabetes. Another 2.2 million deaths were attributable to high blood glucose in 2012**.

- Almost half of all deaths attributable to high blood glucose occurs before the age of 70 years. The WHO estimates that diabetes was the seventh leading cause of death in 2016.

- Healthy diet, regular physical activity, maintaining a normal body weight, and avoiding tobacco use are ways to prevent or delay the onset of type 2 diabetes.

- Diabetes can be treated, and its consequences avoided or delayed with diet, physical activity, medication, and regular screening and treatment for complications.

Alright, now that is done, let us move on. From this point forward, you are going to learn all the skills you need to help you live your healthiest life! Let us do this together.

Health-Happy Meal Ideas

Throughout this book, I will provide some healthy meal options for you to try. Meals are meant to be enjoyed, so try the ones you like, and leave the ones you do not like. What I am aiming to do with these is inspire you to eat less fast food and eat more nourishing meals.

You will also notice that the portion sizes may be smaller than what you are used to. If you need to add more in the beginning, go for it. As you progress through to the end of the book, incrementally reduce the amount of food you put on your plate.

For example, for the first meal suggestion, I am going to share with you one of my favorite meals. It calls for only 2 slices of sweet potato and a handful of string beans with salmon. If you feel you need more, add a couple extra slices of sweet potato, a few more string beans, and a larger portion of salad. The next time you make this meal, cut out the extra sweet potato, and the time after that, cut out the extra beans. But if you are extra hungry on the fourth time, add those sweet potatoes back in, and do not beat yourself up over it.

Not beating yourself up is the key ingredient here! If you are really craving a burger from your favorite fast-food place, it is okay once in a while. Go for it. Just do not do it again the next day. Also, just because you had that burger for lunch, it does not give you a full "cheat day." Get back on track for dinner.

Health-Happy Dinner #1

Main

- 1 slice wild caught salmon
- 2 slices sweet potato
- Handful of steamed string beans

Salad Ingredients

- Romaine lettuce

- Shredded carrots

- Shredded beet roots {optional; not everyone likes beets}

- Sliced radishes

- Sliced cucumber

- 2 tbsp. walnut pieces

- 2 tbsp. washed dried cranberries or raisins

- A few black olives

- 1/4 small red onion

Dressing

- Whisk together:

- 1/2 cup olive oil

- 3 tbsp. lemon Juice

Herbal Tea

CHAPTER 2

Feed Your Health

Enjoy the Food You Eat

"It's easy to impress me. I don't need a fancy party to be happy. Just good friends, good food, and good laughs. I'm happy. I'm satisfied. I'm content."

– Maria Sharapova

2

Love Yourself

Do you love yourself?

It is an honest question. It is one we should ask ourselves often. I understand if you are not the type of person to stand in front of the mirror every day and say, "Hey, I love you." Although, if you are, I think you are doing a great thing. Because when you love yourself, and I mean truly love yourself, you will inevitably treat yourself better.

You will think about the food you put in your body. You will take the time you need to prepare healthier meal options for your day. You will think twice about eating foods that are bad for you. Loving yourself does not mean never allowing yourself to have some of the junk food that you love; it will just stop you from letting it take over your diet completely.

What does loving yourself truly mean?

No two relationships are alike. As with every relationship, it will mean different things to different people. For me, loving myself means putting me first. To some of you, this may sound selfish, but it is not. Putting your needs first, allows you to gain the strength and energy you need to help others.

When you are sending all of your energy out, you are not giving yourself the time to replenish that energy. This is when you become run down, start making unhealthy food choices, stop exercising, and ultimately get sick. When you are sick, you are no good for anyone.

Of course, once in a while, you will need to put your needs behind those of a sick family member, a colleague that could use some help, or a friend in need. But if you are always making the choice to run to the aid of others, I would argue that you do not love yourself enough.

Why?

We procrastinate on the things we do not want to do. It is natural. When you do not love yourself, you do not have an interest in doing the work you need to do to care for yourself, and so you will always make the choice to do something else.

Think about it this way. Remember having homework you didn't want to do? Say, an essay on a topic that bored you to death? What did you do? If you are anything like me, you dusted every single object in your home, and you felt great about your very dust-free home; however, you still had to get that paper done. It did not help with the task, and probably caused added stress as the deadline loomed closer.

How do you know if you love yourself?

There are a few ways:

1. Listen to the words you use to talk to yourself.

2. Think about how often you take the time to do something you love.

3. Observe how you treat your health.

4. Look at how you present yourself to the world.

Listen to the words you use to talk to yourself.

When you make a small mistake, like including a typo in an email, or spilling coffee on your freshly cleaned white shirt, how do you respond? If you are like a large majority of the human population, you will say something like: *I am so stupid,* or *I should have been paying attention,* or *how could I be so dumb?* You think nothing of the strong negative way you view yourself in that insignificant moment, and you go on with the rest of your day. You do not even realize the damage this seemingly small incident is having on your own self-image.

Your brain is amazing. It can change and grow with you as you age, but it will only strengthen the thoughts that you have often. Only you can control those thoughts and create change within yourself. If you often tell yourself how stupid, dumb, ugly, or useless you are, you are strengthening those thought patterns. It is that simple. The best way to strengthen the love you have for yourself is to feed your brain positive thoughts about yourself.

If you find yourself saying mean things to yourself, stop and reframe those thoughts. You can say something like:

Actually, no, I am really smart. That was just a tiny, insignificant mistake that has no real impact on my life.

Or

I am so strong. I handle every challenge that comes my way with confidence.

Or

Wow! I look gorgeous in this outfit.

Talk to yourself the way you talk to others. Would you ever turn to a friend and say: "Wow, you look horrible today!"

Would you look at your grandchild if they dropped their cookie on the floor, and say: "That was stupid! Why would you do that?"

No, you would not. I know you would not. So, why do you allow yourself to do it to you? It is not right. The more you put yourself down, the more negative your self-image will be, and your love for yourself will continue to diminish over time.

Be kind to yourself. Give yourself a break. Reward yourself for a job well done. Tell yourself how great you are every single day. Because you are great. You are always doing the absolute best you can, even on the toughest of days. We all are. BE KIND TO YOURSELF!

Think about how often you take the time to do something you love.

Life is busy. There is always something that needs to be done. There is always someone who needs help. Are you aware of how often you put yourself first in your daily life?

In order to feel happy and free-spirited, you have to take the time to put yourself first and do the things you love. In doing this, you create balance in your life, which in turn gives you the energy to give more to the world around you. But the ultimate goal here is to prove to yourself just how much you love yourself. When you love yourself, you want yourself to feel joy and freedom.

What do you love to do?

Make a list of all the things you love to do. Do not hold yourself back. You can add things that are easy to do daily, and some that you have always wanted to do one day. Make sure to add some things in here that see you getting active! Here is a sample list to give you some inspiration:

1. Light a candle, make a pot of tea, and spend an hour reading for fun.

2. Go hiking.

3. Write a book about your life.

4. Go to a farmer's market.

5. Meet a friend for a coffee or tea.

6. Take a yoga class.

7. Learn how to cook like a chef.

8. Go for a swim at the local community center.

9. Grow a vegetable garden.

10. Take a line dancing class.

11. Take a Zumba class.

12. Go walking.

Observe how you treat your health.

When you stop loving yourself, you will inevitably stop making your own health a priority. Making healthy choices in a world that values convenience and efficiency, can be a challenge. There is always a fast food restaurant on the way home or some quick take-out available.

There is always a reason to skip the physical activity for the day. If you do not love yourself, staying on top of your body's needs will become less and less of a priority. The downward progress can be so gradual that you do not even realize it is happening at first, until one day you are living a life filled with unhealthy habits; habits that reflect your inability to love yourself.

Take a moment and take stock of your current habits. How are you neglecting or even beating your body up? Do you drink a lot of pop or sugary soda? Do you eat a lot of junk food? Do you smoke? How many times a week do you challenge yourself to get active?

You may want to write your assessment down in a journal. But make sure you do not use this as an excuse to beat yourself up. Look at this moment as a beginning. It is the start of your journey to love yourself more. It is a whole new chapter, one where you work every day at loving yourself because you are worth it. In this chapter, we are going to start looking at how you can slowly and meaningfully change your diet to treat yourself and your body with love.

Look at how you present yourself to the world.

Your hygiene is an important indicator. It can tell you a lot about the way you feel about yourself. Do you wear clothes you like and feel great in? What is your cleanliness level? Do you take the time to have a pedicure once in a while? And yes, men, this is a question for you too! Pedicures are so healthy for your feet. Have a pedicure; your feet will thank you!

Of course, there are some days you will leave the house not having worried about brushing your hair, and maybe even having thrown on the rumpled shirt that has been hanging off the chair at the end of your bed. This is completely normal.

Do you ever find yourself saying: "I just do not have time to worry about how I look?"

Or

"What does it matter anyway? I do not care how I look."

These are two very good signs that you need to participate in a whole lot more self-love! The way you present yourself to the world matters. It matters to you and how you see yourself in the world. Open up your closet and have a look at your wardrobe. How much of your clothing do you love and feel great in?

Move those pieces of clothing to be right in the middle of the closet so that they are the first thing you see every single day. Make the choice to wear these clothes more often. Take the time to shower and do your hair. If you wear make-up, put some of your best lipstick on. I promise that even on a grey day, this will lift your mood.

What does loving yourself have to do with managing your diabetes?

Everything! Your journey to a healthier you, even after a diabetes diagnosis, starts with your ability to love yourself. The change to loving yourself more will take more work than you think, but it is the best kind of work; wear clothes you feel great in, get active, take the time to do things you love, and generally just treat yourself with kindness.

Love the Food You Eat

If you were to characterize your relationship with food, what words would you use to describe it? Neglectful? Indifferent? Rushed? Apathetic? Abusive? Or… Loving? Thoughtful? Kind? Caring? Growing? Or a combination of some of the above.

Relationships can be complicated, but they do not have to be. I know that there can be a lot in forming your relationship with food, but I want to ask you one very simple question:

If you loved yourself completely, what words would you use to describe your relationship with food? For me, I would describe my relationship as one that is supportive, nourishing, and of course, loving. It is not like this every day, but it is the ideal I strive for. Having the relationship you want to have with food takes ongoing work. Do not let that discourage you. Once you have a good relationship established, it is a lot easier to maintain.

So, what kind of relationship do you want to have with food, and how does it compare to your current relationship with food? If you feel like you are in an abusive relationship, you may feel like a slave to your cravings. Nothing is ever enough! The sugar monster is always hungry and must be fed. The only problem is that the more you feed it, the stronger it gets.

Let us stop feeding the monster together. There are some people who are great at cutting off the monster's food supply quickly (i.e. quitting pop cold turkey), but I have found that one of the most effective ways to change your relationship, and maintain that change, is to do it slowly and methodically. This means not cutting it all out right away, even though you may be motivated to.

The problem with a strong motivation is that you want instantaneous change. The minute you fail, with this mindset, you immediately beat yourself up and decide you are not strong enough to do it.

Okay, you are right! I should not make assumptions. Some people are great at making drastic change and jumping right back on the wagon if they fall off. More often than not, however, the thing that I have found is that breaking years of habits takes time. Your brain has so much practice leading you to the unhealthy habit choices. I need time to rewire those thought patterns. There are a lot of competing theories on how long it takes to break a habit; I am not here to argue with any of them. The one thing I will say is that I believe it to be an individual process.

Your process is yours and yours alone, so please do what is right for you! I do want to share with you one piece of advice that really helped me love the food I eat.

ENJOY YOUR TIME TOGETHER

It is so simple, right! When you eat, take the time to enjoy the food you are eating. Make it an event rather than a passing thought.

Turn off your computer.

Leave your phone in another room. (Do not worry, the world can wait for you to eat dinner!)

Eat at the dining table with a formal setting. (Basically, do not eat while watching TV.)

Savor each bite. Chew your food. Taste the flavors. Take notice of everything you enjoy. If you have company, be with them in the moment. Let everything on your to-do list go. Share your thoughts, the events of the day… whatever.

Talk, eat, and enjoy.

Taking the time to make your meal an event that allows you to unwind, socialize, and enjoy what you are putting in your body, will inevitably make you feel better.

Stop, take a breath, and eat.

Eat the Food You Love

I know that some of the foods you love are not good for you. It is inevitable. Unhealthy food can be delicious. There is no warning on a quick burger, a chocolate bar, French fries, or a can of pop, that yells, "WAIT! Stop; do not eat this. It is killing you!" When you are starving, your favorite burger is the tastiest thing in this whole world. When you need some sugar to get you through the mid-afternoon energy slump, a can of coke feels like the lift you need. I don't deny it.

But these are not the foods I want you to think about. You probably already think about them every day anyway! The foods I do want you to remember are the healthy foods you love. These are what get lost amongst the easy to get, quick junk food options.

The healthy foods are the ones that are nutrient dense. What exactly does that mean? Nutrient dense foods are ones that contain vitamins, minerals, complex carbohydrates, lean protein, and healthy fats. They are low in calories. Basically, they have a higher ratio of goodness than badness.

According to healthline.com[1], the 11 most nutrient dense foods are:

Salmon
Kale
Seaweed
Garlic
Shellfish
Potatoes
Liver
Sardines
Blueberries
Egg yolks
Dark chocolate

---

1 https://www.healthline.com/health/food-nutrition/sugar-facts-scientific#6

Did you notice that chocolate is on that list? I sure did! Keep in mind as you read this that there will always be conflicting information out there. According to medicalnewstoday.com[2], nuts hit the top of the list. My point here is not to argue who is right and tell you exactly what to eat. I just want to give you some examples of healthy food to help you make healthier choices.

I recently decided to revisit my favorite food list. It changes over time, and I thought it might be a fun idea to actually write out the foods I love. Give it a try for yourself. Choose three of your favorite food groups, and then pick some foods within each group that make your taste buds happy and your body bounce with joy.

Here is my list of the foods that I love:

1. VEGETABLES

I am actually not kidding here. My favorite foods right now are vegetables. It was hard to narrow down which ones, because I really do love a lot of them. For this exercise, I have narrowed it down to romaine lettuce, string beans, and sweet potatoes.

2. FISH

The most delicious fish for me is salmon and red snapper. So good!

---

2 https://www.medicalnewstoday.com/articles/324713.php

3. FRUITS

Again, this was a tough category to cut down, but I managed. The four fruits that made my favorites list are: grapefruit, apples, watermelon with seeds, and pineapple.

The point of this exercise is for you to create a short list of foods that you love, and place it in a spot where you will see it every day, so that when you are feeling the pull to eat badly, you can look at your list and easily choose at least one or two things you really love, to include in your next meal.

How will eating what you love help with your diabetes?

By replacing the bad food with tasty food, which will help you eat better, because you are not missing out on good stuff; you are just changing it. That is all. Your life is still filled with tasty food; you just can not get it at the closest burger joint.

Also, you will start to feel good about yourself, and great about your choices. A higher self-esteem means a whole lot more love for yourself.

You will also notice a change in your weight and a lift in your energy. There are so many amazing reasons to start eating better. The impact of making healthier choices with food is big, and has an effect on all aspects of your life. Start now with the one simple list above. It is not exhaustive or overwhelming, and it can be changed at any time. Write it out and put it on your fridge so that when you are craving a bag of chips, you will have a list of other tasty options right in front of your eyes.

Goodbye Sugar, Hello Results

Sugar is so delicious and so confusing. Some people say you should cut it out altogether; some people say that a certain amount, depending on the amount of calories you eat, is fine. Some people say that sugar is a drug. Some people say that if you eat sugar, you will develop heart disease.

There is also naturally occurring sugar, refined sugar, brown sugar, added sugars… Ahhhhhhhhh…

And the worst thing about sugar is that it is in almost all of the most delicious foods.

What do you do about sugar? First and foremost, listen to the advice of your healthcare practitioner. Everybody is different, and every case is individual. What I will tell you is what I have seen work as an approach to cutting down on sugar. I believe that everything in moderation is doable. I cut out a lot of added sugars, like sugar in my coffee and tea.

This was not an easy task. I used to have at least two teaspoons of sugar in every cup of coffee or tea. That would amount to at least 4 teaspoons a day, 28 teaspoons a week, 112 teaspoons a month, and 1,344 teaspoons a year—just in coffee and tea. That is a lot of sugar! It was an adjustment to get used to coffee without sugar, but I was kind to myself and did it gradually. Little by little, I got used to the flavor of coffee without sugar. You know what I discovered? I did not hate it! And now I actually even really enjoy it.

The other sugary and delicious culprit, which is the cause of so much unnecessary sugar in your body, is—you guessed it—pop! I know that pop can be hard to quit. For some, it's like that morning cup of coffee that gets them going. It might even be your go-to beverage of choice when you sit down to relax for the day. Unfortunately, it is just not good for you.

If you do enjoy pop, how many do you drink in a day?

- If the answer is 3, start by cutting one out every second day.

- When that feels easy, cut out the third pop altogether.

- The next step will be to work on cutting out pop number 2, every second day.

- When that feels easy, cut out the second pop altogether.

- The last and final step will be to say goodbye to your daily pop habit, by cutting out all pop every second day.

- When this feels easy, cut it all out! Goodbye pop, hello better health!

This being said, it is important to remember that if you fall off the wagon, it is okay; just jump right back on. Or, after a while, if you feel like you want to have a pop one day, go for it. If you do go for it, though, remember that it is a one-time, once-in-a-while thing, not a habit!

The more sugar you can let go of in your diet, the better you will feel. Get rid of the sugary drinks altogether, and you will start to notice a significant difference.

Make It Easy

The best way to ensure success is to make it easy on yourself. I know that you are motivated to be better for yourself, but sometimes that just is not enough. There are a few simple ways you can help remove some of the obstacles you may face.

The first one is to remove all of the tempting foods from your home. Finish what you have in the cupboards and then replace what you want to remove from your diet, with a healthier choice from your list. For example, if you love a sugary soda in the evening while watching a movie, replace that with a flavored soda that does not have any sugar added to it. Or if you love to snack on chips, replace those with a bag of mixed nuts.

Let your family know that you will need support along your journey, and ask them to respect the food bans. Who knows, maybe they will feel better for it as well!

The second best way to remove all obstacles is to plan and prepare food ahead of time. It is so easy to quickly grab junk food when we are running from place to place throughout the day. It is hard to find good food when you are in a rush and your stomach is growling at you. So set yourself up for success by making a lunch that includes a few snacks, either the night before or prior to leaving in the morning.

A few great suggestions for easy to make and pack foods are: egg salad sandwiches, boiled eggs, quinoa salad with veggies, and fruits.

Manage Your Mindset

In this chapter, you have already begun to work on how you engage with food in your daily life, by:

1. Loving yourself.

2. Having a healthy relationship with food.

3. Reducing your sugar intake in a manageable way.

4. Replacing unhealthy choices with healthy ones, by remembering the good foods that taste good.

I want to give you some affirmations to help you rewire your brain for success. As we have already talked about, your thoughts have a lot of power over the choices you make. If you have never worked with affirmations before, this may feel just as silly as it would to look in the mirror and say *I love you* out loud. Either way, I will leave these here for you to decide what to do with it.

Instructions:

You can either write these out in your journal every morning before starting your day, record them and listen to them at least once a day, or fold this page and read them to yourself at least once a day.

It does not really matter how you take them in; all that matters is that you do it consistently, if you choose to take on this exercise. Also, work with affirmations that make you feel something when you read them. If they do not work for you, reword them so that they do, or do not bother with them at all.

Affirmations:

1. For loving yourself:

   - I love everything about myself.

   - I accept myself for who I am.

   - The best thing about being me is _____.

2. For having a healthy relationship with food:

   - Healthy food makes me happy.

   - I love my body and, therefore, I give it the nutrients it needs.

   - I love good food, and good food loves me.

3. For reducing sugar:

   - I have all the energy I need to have a great day.

   - My health matters.

   - I love myself and I love feeling great.

4. For making healthy choices:

   - I make smart choices with food.

   - I take my health seriously.

   - I value my life.

Health-Happy Breakfast #1

- 1 small bowl of mixed fruits

- 1 boiled egg

- 1 bowl of oats porridge with almond milk {no sugar}

- Coffee or herbal tea {no sugar}

CHAPTER 3

Get Moving

Get Happy

"True enjoyment comes from the activity of the mind, and exercise of the body; the two are ever united."

– Wilhelm von Humboldt

3

WALK, WALK, WALK

Did you know that for most people, there is not much more energy spent in running a kilometer than there is in walking it? The only real difference is that walking takes longer. When I first read that, I was surprised. I most certainly thought running would take much more energy.

In my younger years, I did not think much of walking as a form of exercise. It was just the thing I did to get from one place to another. I discounted it because it did not feel like I was doing anything difficult. But walking is actually one of the best and most healthy ways to remain physically active as we age.

There are a few reasons for this:

1. **You can walk anywhere.** Put on some comfortable shoes, open the front door, and away you go. If the weather is bad, you can walk around your home. When I say this though, I mean that you take the time and make your walking intentional. Set a goal; something like, "I will walk from my dining room to the front door 20 times, take a 5-minute break, and then do the same thing again.

2. **It does not cost anything.** You probably already own a comfy pair of shoes that you can use for a good walk. There is no need to buy expensive yoga pants, unless of course you like them. You do not even need any fancy protective gear, like a helmet. All you need is you, your desire to feel great, and the clothes you would normally wear anyway.

3. **You can do it on your own time.** No need to check your schedule or move things around to fit a class in; no need to cancel your coffee date with the girls; no need to worry about whether or not you will be able to get to an appointment on time after you run from the gym—the only thing you need to do, and this is a very important one, is to MAKE WALKING A PRIORITY. That is all. It is that easy.

4. **It is low maintenance.** You do not have to worry about packing anything. All you need is you!

Here are some answers to common questions people have when developing a walking routine, when they have not had one before or for a really long time:

1. How often should you walk?

The easy answer here is, every single day for 30 minutes. Research has found that:

"Just 30 minutes every day can increase cardiovascular fitness, strengthen bones, reduce excess body fat, and boost muscle power and endurance. It can also reduce your risk of developing conditions such as heart disease, type 2 diabetes, osteoporosis, and some cancers."[3]

I started off this chapter on the importance of exercise with walking, because it is one of the easiest and cost effective ways to stay active every single day. Exercise does not have to be complicated or expensive. Make it easy, and just keep doing it. Believe me, your body will thank you for it for years to come.

If you have got a lot on your plate and find it hard to carve out 30 minutes every day, do not give up altogether. Every little bit helps—5 days a week, 3 days a week, or 1 day a week—whatever you can do, will help you. That being said, if you are truly committed to your health, you will make walking a priority, and hopefully find the 30 minutes at least 5 days every week.

2. What if I find that walking for 30 minutes is difficult?

Do not beat yourself up!
Do not use it as an excuse to not try!
Do not let your low physical fitness bring you down!

---

3 https://www.betterhealth.vic.gov.au/health/healthyliving/walking-for-good-health

Everyone starts somewhere. If you do not start, you will never get better; in fact, you will only get worse. As we age, it does get harder. That is a simple fact of life. So be kind to your body! Begin your walking routine by taking shorter walks. Here is a simple pattern for building up your endurance:

Week 1 – Take three 5-minute walks a day, with at least a 30-minute break in between each. You can also spread the walks out, to work with your schedule.

Week 2 – Take one 5-minute walk and two 10-minute walks a day, with at least a 30-minute break in between each. You can also spread the walks out, to work with your schedule.

Week 3 – Take three 10-minute walks a day, with at least a 30-minute break in between each. You can also spread the walks out, to work with your schedule.

Week 4 – Take three 10-minute walks a day, with only a 5-minute break in between each.

Week 5 – Take one 20-minute walk a day, without any breaks.

Week 6 – Take one 30-minute walk a day, without any breaks.

This breakdown of building yourself up to walking for 30 minutes a day is a suggestion to get you thinking about what works for you. If you find that three 10-minute walks a day feels really good, you can do that for much longer than a week, before moving to the next stage. If you can not go longer than a 5-minute walk for a month, that is okay. Keep going. Keep pushing for more until it feels good. Do what works for you and for your body.

It is never too late to take your health seriously. If you feel like you have gone past the point of being helped, you are wrong. It is never too late to start!

What pace should I walk at?

Can you guess what I am going to say here? Probably! But I am going to say it anyway: DO WHAT WORKS BEST FOR YOU!

That said, a general rule of thumb is that you should not be so out of breath that you can not speak, but you should be walking fast enough that you can not sing.

Always listen to your body. I know you are motivated to feel better, and so you may force yourself to push through any pain, but sometimes pain is a warning sign. If you are feeling pain that goes beyond the general soreness you would feel from moving muscles that you normally do not use, then stop. See a doctor and find out what is wrong. Sometimes pain is telling you that you need insoles, or that you need to ease into your new exercise regime. The bottom line is always to listen to your body.

No More Excuses!

If you have a million different reasons as to why you can not get active, then I am so glad you are here. This book is exactly what you need for kicking your behind into action. Today is the day you are going to start. Do not wait. Start right now. Put this book down and go for a walk, either around your house or around the block. Start with five minutes.

Do not worry, I am not going anywhere. I will be right here when you get back. If you are thinking, "Well, no, I always finish a whole chapter before I put a book down," and this is stopping you, it is just an excuse! You heard me. You are allowing yourself to procrastinate. Do not get me wrong; I am really glad you have made my book a priority, but in this very moment, I want you to redirect your priority to being more physically active. Now go. Get up off the couch and get moving!

...Hey, you are back! See, I told you I had still been here. How did it go? Take a moment and congratulate yourself for a job well done. You did it! You started. You had the courage to begin your journey to becoming more physically active and ultimately healthier. How did it feel?

As you continue along your own personal path to better health, you will have to fight against the multitude of excuses you will tell yourself. Some of the most common are:

- I can not do it! I am too out of shape.

- I will make things worse by hurting myself.

- I have never been very fit, so why start now?

- Working out is boring.

- I am way too busy.

- I am so tired. It will not do me any good.

- I play with the grandkids; is not that enough?

- I move my body a lot when I am cleaning the house.

And the most common of all the common excuses to ever be uttered by every single human being on this planet: I WILL DO IT TOMORROW!

How many of those excuses have you said, either to yourself or someone else in your life? I am going to guess that you have said at least five of those excuses. Starting today, you are going to take the power away from your excuses. Yes, there will be the odd day when you are actually too busy with activities that are really important to you. That is 100% okay. You just have to make sure that a day like this only happens once in a blue moon.

How do you take the power away from your excuses?

Excuses are motivated by a few different factors:

1. A desire to remain in your comfort zone

2. Fear of change

3. Worry over what others will think

A desire to remain in your comfort zone:

When you do something over and over and over again, for years of your life, your brain and body expect that you will keep following that same pattern. It is easy. It is comfortable. It is what they know. It is what you know.

It is only natural that you will meet some resistance when you try to push yourself out of your comfort zone. Your brain needs to create new thought patterns. It is like going on a hike and choosing to make your own way through the forest, even though there is a perfectly good, well-travelled path. It is harder. You will not get where you are going as quickly. You will have to think on your feet.

Physically, you are comfortable doing what you always do. Your body is used to the way you move, even if it is not in its best shape. It will take work to change it, and that work may hurt. Your muscles will ache as you begin to put them to work. What do you think would happen? Your muscles have been napping for years, and now, all of a sudden, you want them to work for you! Of course you will meet some painful resistance. This is okay.

Listen to your body and be kind to it. Thank it for its work, with a warm bath and some delicious, healthy food. And then get back up off the couch and try again and again and again, until your body is more comfortable being active than it is being sedentary.

Fear of change:

When you push yourself out of your comfort zone, you will need to confront your fear of change. If you are thinking, "Why would I be afraid of getting healthy?" take a moment and think about why you stopped being active in the first place. This is where your answer lies. The answer will be different for everyone. But in some way, fear always informs your reasoning. Whether you were afraid to put your needs above those of others because you were fearful of being selfish, or you were afraid of not succeeding in achieving the goal you set for yourself, it does not matter. Fear is fear, and you have to get to the bottom of it to move forward.

Fear expertly hides itself within our excuses. So start this process by thinking about all of the excuses you have given in order to get out of being active, and then find the fear that is forming here.

Here are a few examples to get you started:

1. **Excuse**
   I do not have time.

   Fear
   I will not be able to help my kids and my grandkids enough. They need me. I can't let them down.

2. **Excuse**
   I hate going to the gym.

   Fear
   I will fail and look stupid.

3. **Excuse**
   Whenever I pay for a membership or group of classes, I waste money because I stop going.

   Fear
   I do not have the discipline to stick with a program. I do not want to feel bad about myself, so I just will not try.

The next step is to let those fears know that they do not need to protect you anymore. Try something like this:

1. **Excuse**
   I do not have time.

   Fear
   I will not be able to help my kids and my grandkids enough. They need me. I can't let them down.

   Response
   THANK YOU *FEAR* FOR HAVING MY BEST INTEREST AT HEART. BUT I KNOW THAT THE BETTER I FEEL, THE MORE I CAN DO FOR MY FAMILY. TAKING THE TIME TO PUT MY HEALTH FIRST DOES NOT MAKE ME SELFISH.

2. **Excuse**
   I hate going to the gym.

   Fear
   I will fail and look stupid.

   Response
   I HEAR YOU *FEAR*. FAILING IS HARD AND FEELS UNCOMFORTABLE, BUT SOMETIMES IT IS NECESSARY. IF I FAIL ONE DAY, I'LL SUCCEED THE NEXT.

3. **Excuse**

   Whenever I pay for a membership or group of classes, I waste money because I stop going.

   Fear

   I do not have the discipline to stick with a program. I do not want to feel bad about myself, so I just will not try.

   Response

   YES, *FEAR*, IT MAY LOOK LIKE I DO NOT HAVE THE DISCIPLINE, BUT THE ACTUAL FACT IS THAT I HAVE NOT FOUND THE THING THAT I LOVE TO DO YET. I AM GOING TO KEEP WORKING ON IT.

Basically, you need to understand why you are making the excuses you are, address the fear behind them, and then move forward with a positive solution. You can do this! Do not let your fears stand in your way. The change that you crave is for the better. By being active and achieving greater physical fitness, you will see your quality of life get better with time. That is worth so much more than your fear and its desire to leave you comfortably sitting in your comfy armchair every day.

Worry over what others will think:

Change may be easy for you to take on, but it may be hard for your loved ones and friends to accept. Of course, they do not want to see you unhealthy; and of course, they want to see you happy, but they may struggle with the changing version of you that they know and love.

Your changes may also affect their lives in ways they were not ready for yet. For example, you taking a more proactive approach to your health, may make them question their own choices. This questioning will make them face the fact that they too have been neglecting their health as well. Sometimes when people are forced to confront a reality they do not want to, they may lash out at the person forcing them to do it. This is their issue, not yours. You have to do what is best for you.

Another worry that often stops people from going to the gym or signing up for a class, is that they will look stupid in front of the more fit people. Yes; in the beginning, it may be obvious to others that you are struggling. There are two important things to remember here: Most often, people are too focused on themselves to pay any attention to you and how you are doing; and if they are looking at you and judging, it is because they have self-confidence issues that they need to address. Any outside judgement that is coming your way has absolutely nothing to do with you!

It is really important to remember that last point:

The judgement of others has nothing to do with you.

Your health is all about you. YOU are actually the one and only person who matters when it comes to your health. It is that simple. It is all about YOU and what YOU need. So stop worrying about what others think.

You can ask for advice from professionals. You can ask for support from your loved ones and friends. You can let everyone in your life know that the positive changes you are making in your life are for you. They may support you in the ways that you need to succeed, and they may not—it does not matter. You have to find the strength within to stand strong on your own, because:

YOU MATTER.

TRY, TRY, & TRY Again

How often in your life have you thought to yourself that you would love to take either a dance class, a yoga class, or a running class, and then you go a few times, and then never, ever go back. When you decide to skip a class for whatever thing you have decided was more important that day, you thought to yourself: "It is okay if I miss one; I will go back next week."

But then next week rolls around, and you have lost your momentum. You are really busy, and there are so many other things you could accomplish in the time it would take you to pack up your things, drive to the class, take the class, shower after the class, and wash your workout clothes for next time.

"It is okay," you tell yourself. "I can catch up next week. There are still six more classes left this session. It will be fine."

But then next week rolls around again, and you realize everyone will be so far ahead of you. You start to think about how embarrassing it would be if the class is held up because you do not know what you are doing and can not keep up. So you do not go. You think maybe you will try again the following week, but deep down, you know you will not.

This has happened to me so many times. I have signed up for multiple gym memberships, only to completely stop going within a couple of months. I have tried Curves, and let go of that too. I have signed up for dance classes that I have never finished. I have stopped myself from signing up for these same classes the following term because I told myself I had failed just like I did the last time.

The weird thing is that I want to be healthy, and I know that staying physically active is a big part of that, and yet sometimes I still could not bring myself to go. Why? Like we have been talking about in this chapter, I allowed myself to listen to the excuses I was telling myself, but sometimes it was actually because the program or class did not suit either my needs or my schedule.

It is all fine and good to push yourself, but be realistic.

If you sign up for an advanced class when you are not ready, you are setting yourself up for failure.

If you sign yourself up for a class at 6 am because you want to push yourself, but you actually hate early mornings, you are setting yourself up for failure.

If you pay for a gym membership even though you have no desire to run on a treadmill, lift a weight, or hire a trainer to teach you how to use the equipment, you are setting yourself up for failure.

If you decide that you are going to do everything alone because you do not want anyone you know to see you struggling, but you know you are more motivated when you have company, you are setting yourself up for failure.

Do not set yourself up for failure. Yes, there will be something you try that will not work for you. This is not a failure; this is trial and error. But if you know for sure that something does not work for you—such as running makes your knees hurt—for goodness sake, do not do it! I do not regret having tried the things that did not work for me, because now I know more about what I want.

So keep on trying things until you find the things that you love and get you excited. Try, try, and try again, until you get it right!

Activities That Get You Active

Sometimes it can be hard to think up something new to try. So I made a list of some fun activities that will get you moving. Remember that it does not have to be so hard that you cringe when you think of doing it, and it also does not have to be super-fast. You just need to be moving your body.

One thing that helps is if it is fun! Here are some activities that I find fun:

- Line dancing
- Swimming
- Aquafit
- Walking with a friend
- Bowling
- Tennis

- Yoga

- Ballroom dancing

- Putting on my favorite music and dancing around the house

Remember that just because I like doing these activities, does not mean you will! Take a moment and think of at least five different activities you could incorporate into your life that will help you stay committed to being more physically active on a daily basis.

Set Yourself up for Success

One of the best ways you can set yourself up for success is to make sure the activities you choose are not boring. If you cringe at the thought of whatever it is you have signed yourself up to do, you will be less likely to go when life presents you with other options. So do the things you love doing. Take the list you just wrote of the five activities you want to try, and put them in your schedule. If some of those things require you to sign up, google the available options in your area, or talk to some friends in your community to see if anyone has any suggestions.

Be aware of your current level of physical fitness, and do not push yourself too far beyond what you are capable of right away. If it feels like torture, you and your body will find every excuse possible to not subject yourself to it on a regular basis. Start at a reasonable level, one where you are pushing yourself but at a manageable pace. If you push yourself too hard, too fast, you also run the risk of injuring your body, which will set you back even further.

Enlist a family member or friend to be your exercise buddy. There are so many benefits to having an exercise buddy, but the two most important are that you get to catch up with someone you love spending time with, and you have an accountability partner who will help keep you on track.

Find an expert to inspire you. For me, when I was trying to walk in my home during the winter months, I found myself putting it off all day until I just did not do it. One of the things that inspired me to do it was a walking video. I would put it on, and off I went. There was something about having someone there (well, sort of) to inspire me to keep pushing forward that made me do it.

Do not compare yourself to anyone else, ever! Your journey is yours and yours alone. It does not matter what anyone else in the world is doing—not the woman beside you in yoga, with her legs behind her head; not the neighbor who lost an extra 10 pounds last month; and not the guy who ran a half-marathon at the age of 106. You are you, and you will do amazing as long as you just start and, no matter what, find a way to keep going.

If you fall off the boat, there will always be a rope to help you back on. It is never too late to be more active!

Do what you love.
Start slowly.
Listen to your body.
LOVE YOURSELF!

Build a Program That Works for You

Like I said earlier, it is recommended that you move your body in some way every single day, but I understand that sometimes life gets in the way. The thing to always remember is that this is absolutely okay, as long as you are still making some form of physical fitness a priority, at least three to four days a week.

One of the things I have found is that once you get in the habit of exercising, you will want to do more of it, so you will find a way to get in a fifteen-minute walk, even on the busiest of days.

Here are a few tips when creating a schedule of activities that will work best for you:

1. Choose activities that you like.

2. Add at least two different activities. For example, line dancing and walking, or walking and bowling.

3. Make sure to choose the days and times when other obligations most likely will not get in the way.

4. Schedule your activities at a time that works for you. If you feel tired in the evening, try to join an afternoon class or go for your walk in the morning.

5. If you do not enjoy something after trying it for a while, do not stubbornly hold onto it. Let it go. It is okay. Try something else instead!

Walking with My Sister

During one of my sister's first visits after she was diagnosed with diabetes, we began walking together. She could barely walk and had a really hard time keeping up. She would always end up trailing behind me, and I would have to stop to let her catch up.

But I kept inspiring her to join me, and she stayed motivated by her desire to feel better. One night, on a later visit, I had not expected her to have made such good progress. I thought I was way ahead of her, but when I turned around to see where she was, she was right in my face. I was so proud of how much she had accomplished.

You can do it too. All you have to do is take your health seriously. When you do, and you keep at it, you will start to see progress too.

Walking Tip

Recently, I found a video that I love. It helps me to get active at home whenever I have the time. It also really helps during the winter months when it can be more difficult, or dangerous, to walk outside. It helps that the video is also really fun to walk with. If you need a little inspiration to get active in your home, check out this link: https://youtu.be/X3q5e1pV4pc.

The Bottom Line

Moving your body is good for you. If you do not keep moving, you will lose your ability to move altogether. Better physical fitness has so many benefits:

1. You will have less pain when you do need to move.

2. You will feel better about yourself.

3. You will lose weight.

4. You will improve your circulation.

5. You may see your blood sugar levels become more regulated.

6. You may also experience an increased sensitivity in your body to insulin.

7. You will raise your body's healthy HDL cholesterol.

8. You will reduce your anxiety.[4]

Health-Happy Lunch #1

Salad

- Mixed leafy greens

- 1/4 cup mushrooms diced

- 1/3 red onion, chopped

- 1/4 cup diced zucchini

- 1/2 cup sliced cucumber and radishes

- Diced red, yellow, and orange pepper

- A few black olives

---

4 https://www.health.harvard.edu/staying-healthy/the-importance-of-exercise-when-you-have-diabetes

Dressing

Blend together:

- ¼ cup Styrian pumpkin seed oil

- 2 tbsp sesame paste

- Sliced sun-dried tomatoes

- Pinch of cumin and salt

CHAPTER 4

Hygiene for Happiness

*Taking Care of Yourself
Can Improve Your Life*

*"Self-care is never a selfish act—
it is simply good stewardship of
the only gift I have, the gift
I was put on earth to offer
to others."*

– Parker Palmer

4

Look Good, Feel Great

It is time now to talk about the thing we all really do not want to talk about because, well, it is awkward. Have you ever been out with a friend and, in all honesty, they smelled bad—and not just a little bit bad either?

There is a big part of you that wants to say something because you know that they may not even realize it. You think to yourself that you should talk to them about it and ask if they are okay, but you chicken out. What if they get embarrassed? What if they avoid going out with you again in the future? What if they never, ever talk to you again? What if you make them feel so bad that they stop going out altogether?

But then again, now you have just let your friend wander around in public smelling badly?

Either way, you do not feel good about it. Consider me your friend. This chapter of this book is my way of saying to you: "If you are not showering on a regular basis, you probably smell."

There you go. I said it. It is out in the open. Now what are we going to do about it?

We are going to talk about your personal hygiene and how it can affect your health, of course! My promise to you is that I will do my very best to keep it quick and, if possible, fun.

When you are not taking care of your physical cleanliness, it is often a sign that something else is going on. I do not think anyone truly enjoys the feeling of being unclean. First of all, it is physically uncomfortable; and second of all, it can be socially isolating. I have never met anyone in my life who wakes up in the morning and says, "I am going to enjoy staying dirty today!"

So, what are some of the things poor hygiene can be an indicator of?

1. Low mood
2. Poor self-esteem
3. Lack of self-love
4. No energy
5. Physical barriers to bathing regularly
6. Depression
7. Dementia

Hygiene is not just about bathing or showering; it is also about your overall appearance. Is your hair brushed? Does it need a trim or even a good cut? Are your nails trimmed and clean? Do you need a shave?

The cleanliness of your clothing also has a lot to do with how you feel about the way you look. If your clothes are stained or do not fit well, you may not feel great about being out in public. It is not vain to care about how you present yourself to the world. It is normal. A big part of how we feel socially can have to do with how we look. I am not talking about being a supermodel and spending hours on your make-up, unless that is what you love to do. I am talking about feeling great in your skin and in your clothes.

When we are feeling down, it can be hard to take care of our appearance. It can start slowly: missing a shower one day, deciding to not wash your hair for a fourth day, putting on a shirt you have worn for the last two days because *it does not seem too bad.*

Once you slide down that slippery slope, it can be overwhelming to climb back up. Let us start with one small step at a time. Even if you feel good about your personal hygiene, this short chapter may give you a few tips to help make the process a little easier.

What's in Your Closet?

Dress to impress... yourself! You are the only person who needs to feel good about your wardrobe, and not just good but amazing! I know, some days it is easy to throw on anything that covers your body in a comfortable way, but it can actually bring you down even more.

You may think your clothing does not have anything to do with your mood, but it actually has a lot to do with it. Like I said above, it can be an indicator of depression, but it can also bring you even further down. If you are already beating yourself up, when you look in the mirror and do not like what you see, you will beat yourself up even more.

Let us start by taking a peek into your closet.

Are you still sitting, reading this book? That is not the way to do it. When I say, let us take a peek in your closet, I mean let us actually get up, go into your bedroom, and open the closet door.

Do not forget to bring me with you!

Are you ready?

Great!

STEP 1

The first task is a very easy one! All you have to do is remove any items that are stained or have holes in them. If you saved the ones with holes because you thought you were going to have them mended, but it has been more than six months and you have not done it yet, throw them out. Seriously, let them go!

The same goes for the ones with stains; if you have been saving them to wear around the house, do not. How you feel at home is just as important to your mental health as how you feel out in the world. Save one shirt and one pair of pants for the dirty tasks like cleaning, yard work, or painting, but let the rest go. You do not need them, and you should not be wearing them.

Why?

Wearing stained or ruined clothing can have a negative effect on how you feel about yourself, whether you realize it or not. From this day forward, you are making a promise to yourself to wear clothes that make you feel good. Ruined clothing does not do that!

STEP 2

This step will take a little longer, so if you cannot commit to completing this today, I understand. What I do suggest is that you commit to getting this done by the end of the week. My challenge for you is: Try on everything that is hanging up in your closet, by the end of the week, and decide whether or not you are going to keep it or let it go.

Here are a few things to think about when making your decision:

1. **Do I like how this fits my body?** Our bodies, as you know, are ever changing. The way a piece of clothing sits on your body can make or break how you feel about how you look that day. The truth is, sometimes a piece of clothing that you love, just does not love you. Let it go! Keep the pieces that make you feel good in your body, and that hug all the right spots.

2. **Can I move in it?** This is an important one for me. Does a piece of clothing hinder your ability to walk or sit comfortably? If so, let it go! Your body needs to move.

3. **Do I still like the style?** Remember that you can always redefine your style. You do not even have to consider yourself stylish to do it! I do believe it is important to wear clothes that you like. In this moment, do …

STEP 3

GO SHOPPING! Now, before you slam the book shut, you may be thinking: *Pauline, what do you think I am? Rich?*

My honest answer here is that I do not know. I have absolutely no idea if you can afford a whole new wardrobe or not. My advice is to spend what you personally can afford, and buy yourself at least two new pieces of clothing that you love and feel great in.

This may require some time and thought. Do not just pick any old thing off the shelf. Walk through stores you never go in. Really look. If shopping is not your favorite thing to do, bring a friend and make it fun. They also might be able to help you think outside the box, and get you out of your fashion comfort zone.

The bottom line: Wear clothes that make you feel alive, energetic, and ready for the day. Your style, even if it is not runway ready (99.9999999% of us do not even understand the things that people wear on the runway!), will help you engage with your daily activities with more confidence and pride.

Your Daily Hygiene Routine

From birth, we have a daily hygiene routine. As we get older, we find the things that work best for us. If you are currently not happy with the level of hygiene you are able to maintain, I recommend establishing a routine that is manageable for you.

For me, personally, there are many benefits to having a shower in the morning daily. You do not have to wash your hair every day, but a full body wash serves to help me feel fresh, awake, and ready for the day. My hair does not need a daily wash, so I aim to give it a shampoo at least three times a week.

I trim my fingernails at least once a week, but if you like to keep your nails a little longer, you can always just file them once a week. Keeping your toenails trimmed and clean is so important. Generally, toenails get thicker as we age, making them more difficult to cut; so if you do not keep on top of it, they can become unmanageable. I try to clean and trim them at least once a week.

Here is a sample hygiene routine:

MONDAY
Morning shower
Shampoo hair

TUESDAY
Morning shower

WEDNESDAY
Morning shower
Trim toenails and clean feet thoroughly

THURSDAY
Morning shower
Shampoo hair

FRIDAY
Morning shower
Trim fingernails

SATURDAY
Have a relaxing bath and shave legs

SUNDAY
Morning shower

MONTHLY
Every 6 months (or more), go to the salon for a haircut

I know this seems really simple, and I know you probably do not need to see this. Yes, it is easy to come up with a schedule, and you probably could have done it on your own without me giving you an example. Sometimes we need a simple reminder. Even me. Even you.

On a fresh sheet of paper, print out the week days, and create a hygiene schedule for yourself. Hang it in a place in your home where you will see it as a regular reminder to stay on top of your hygiene. On the days when you find yourself making the "I will do it tomorrow" excuse, you will see that reminder and know that you cannot take two showers to make up for it. It is on the list, so get it done today!

The Pros and Cons of a Professional Pedicure

Pedicures are often one of those luxuries we indulge in to get our feet looking fine during the summer months. We agonize over the next fun color. Will it match our sandals? Will it clash with what I usually wear? We sit in the chair and relax as a skilled esthetician massages the tension out of our calves. It is always such a nice treat!

Pedicures, however, can pose a problem for those who have diabetes, because they are at risk of complications. There can be a lot of bacteria swimming around in that water if the spa is not careful. Also, if you have a cut, or obtain a cut while at the spa, you put yourself at risk of getting an infection, which is never good.

That being said, a pedicure can work wonders for your feet. Having a professional take the time to really clean and hydrate your feet can help keep you complication free. So, how do you know when you should go to a spa for a pedicure[5]?

1. **If you are not complication free, do not go!**
   This means if you have an ulcer, infection, cut, or neuropathy, do not risk it. The pedicure is not worth the potential for further complications.

---

5 http://www.diabetesforecast.org/2008/jul/the-truth-about-pedicures.html

2. **Research the spa.** Read reviews online, or call and ask what their cleaning procedures are. If the spa does not know exactly, then do not risk it. Do not just turn up at a strip mall salon and see if you get a good feeling.

3. **Have a look at the foot bath.** Bacteria can live in the pipes, so try to find a spa near you that has a pipeless tube.

4. **Ask, when booking, if they work differently with clients who have diabetes.** If they are not sure, this is not the spa for you. The estheticians should know to go lighter on the massage, and to be extra careful not to cause any cuts or abrasions.

I know this sounds like a lot of work, but once you have found a great spa that understands how important it is to be careful with your feet, you will never have to do the initial work again. If you cannot find any that you feel comfortable with, look for a chiropodist in your area. They will understand how to maintain your foot care, and will have experience working with the needs of those with diabetes. You may even be able to find one that will come to your house.

Maintain Your Independence

"The trouble is, when a number—your age— becomes your identity, you've given away your power to choose your future."

– Richard J. Leider

It can be hard to admit that we need help. Our bodies change with each year, and the worst thing you can do is to not admit to yourself that you need some assistance. One of the main reasons people begin to lose control of their daily hygiene routine is due to a lack of confidence getting in and out of or standing in the shower.

You know when your balance does not feel the same as it used to. The best thing to do is to just admit it already! Stop hindering yourself, and start making things easier for you to live life fully. One of the best ways to do this is to have an occupational therapist assess your bathroom and your needs. It does not take long. A new bar here, another bar there, or even a seat to get you through a nice, long shower, will not hurt. In fact, it will save you from either breaking a bone or letting your hygiene go.

Keep your confidence in the shower high, by putting the supports in that you need in order to help yourself, because the other options will see you losing the independence you aim to hold onto.

Rediscover How Great It Feels to Look Good

Maintaining your personal hygiene does take a little bit of work, but it is worth it! Looking good and feeling clean has the ability to lift your mood. It will also ensure that you never miss an opportunity to go out into the world because you did not have the energy to do it all in one day. Keeping your feet clean and complication free will also help your mood and energy stay high.

There are so many benefits to looking your best. You are worth it. Your life is worth it. Take the time you need in order to feel great about yourself!

Health-Happy Dinner #2

Small bowl of light chicken soup
Roasted chicken

Quinoa salad
Ingredients: quinoa; diced red, yellow, and orange peppers; diced cucumber; red onion; and chopped parsley

Dressing: olive oil, pumpkin seed oil, lime juice, pinch of cumin salt, and pepper to taste

Steamed mixed vegetables
Small glass of carrot juice

Dessert: a small slice of no-sugar, no-egg banana bread/ cake

Herbal tea or coffee

CHAPTER 5

Support Your Health

Get Help from Your Family and Friends

"Strong people don't put others down... They lift them up."

– Michael P. Watson

5

Raise Your Self-Esteem

self-es·teem
/'͵self ə'stēm/
noun

1. confidence in one's own worth or abilities; self-respect.

If you think back over your life, when were the times when you felt the best about yourself? Was it after receiving positive marks in school? Or when you finished a marathon you never thought you could run in a thousand years? Or was it when you got the job you had been working so hard for?

While failure can knock your self-esteem down a peg, success has the powerful ability to lift you up. Your self-worth is dependent on your own unique list of criteria. What you feel is valuable about yourself as a person, others may not desire in themselves. For example, I strive to inspire others to care for their bodies and live the healthiest life possible. I love myself for having the ability and the courage to do this, but when I have those days when I cannot do it for myself, it takes my self-esteem down.

I pride myself on getting up each day with the intention to live as fully as I can. But there are days when I just want to stay in bed and pull the covers up over my head. In all honesty, it is not because I really want to; I just feel down and overwhelmed by life, so it is more that I actually cannot get out of bed. They do not happen too often, but when they do, I struggle to be kind to myself. My confidence in my own worth takes a bit of a hit. I am human. I make mistakes. I cry. I get frustrated with the challenges this life throws my way. But I do not give up.

One of the best tools you can add to your collection as you continue to build a stronger you, is the support of family and friends. Think about carrying an awkwardly long but not too heavy box into the house from the driveway. You could probably do it. In fact, you know you could do it without hurting yourself but that it would be a struggle to get it through the front door. Then your neighbor notices you and offers to help.

You could do one of two things: say "no" and stubbornly struggle with the box yourself, or say "yes" and have a much easier time of it.

What happens if that neighbor is out front, but they do not ask, and you don't have the type of relationship where you feel like you could ask them for help? Is there someone at home that you could ask?

I think you get my point. If there is something you could use some help with, seek out the help you need. Do not carry the uncomfortable weight on your own. The same goes with your self-esteem. If you feel like your self-esteem could use a boost, enlist the help of a family member, friend, or community.

The Role of Health in High Self-Esteem

Loss, failure, and abuse are only a few of the challenges we face in life that can cause a lower self-esteem. But I have found one of the biggest blows comes as we age, and our bodies can no longer do the things we once did.

"I am so stupid."

"I am so weak."

"I used to be able to remember the names of everyone I met."

"I used to be able to run 21K."

Add a diabetes diagnosis on top of that, and your self-worth can feel like it is at an all-time low. If you are experiencing this now, do not carry the weight on your own. Find the support you need.

The best place to find that support is in your home, with your family. They are with you more than anyone else, and they know you better than anyone else. That said,

I know that sometimes it is not possible to get help at home. You may live alone, or the family that does live with you is unable to support you due to their own failing health, or they are simply unwilling to support you in your lifestyle change because that might mean they would also have to address their own unhealthy habits. If either of these sounds like a situation you are facing, there are still options; you never have to go it alone.

The first and most obvious option is to seek the support of friends, and the second is to join a program or community center where you can meet new people. I know that some of you reading this may be thinking, "No, I do not have any of that available to me." A range of excuses may come to mind:

1. My friends are busy dealing with their own troubles.

2. I do not have close friends.

3. I do not know anyone who would want to support me.

4. I am not very social.

5. I am not a joiner.

I am here to remind you that these are excuses. There is always a network of support you can access. If you cannot think of any, talk to your doctor; they might be able to suggest a therapist you can talk to, or a local group. Sometimes it helps to meet with others who have also recently been diagnosed with diabetes, and there may be a Meetup in your area.

There is always an option. You just need to look for it. Finding support is a key element to your success in achieving better health. Do not put it aside; find the help you need today! Seriously, today!

Communicate Your Needs and Feelings

"Communication is the solvent of all problems and is the foundation for personal development."

– Peter Shepherd

How many times have you heard, "Communication is key," or "The key to a good relationship is good communication," or …? I imagine you have heard at least one version of something like either of these, more times than you can count in your life. I know I have.

It makes communication sound simple, but I do not think it is as simple as these one-liners lead us to believe. It can be, but at times it can also be complicated. It is good to recognize it and not let it stop you. Always remember that asking for help can always be met with a "no." That is 100% okay. Everyone has boundaries. But if it is family, you then have to find a way to make it clear that your life depends on it, and then maybe you can come to a compromise.

Where Do You Start?

The best place to start is with your diagnosis, prognosis, and what you need to do to maintain good health with diabetes. You should be completely honest with your family member. They need to know exactly what you are going through, how you are feeling about it, and how you are hoping they can help you.

From there, you need to listen too. They love you; they are your family, and your diagnosis will have an impact on them as well. So make sure to ask how they are feeling too.

Get the Help You Need

Make sure to be really clear about the kind of support you are looking for from your family. Be fair in what you ask for though. Remember that the more you do for yourself, the better off you will be.

There are three main areas of support where your family can offer ongoing support:

1. **Lend an ear, and a shoulder.**

   Ask your loved ones to be there for you when you need to talk about all that you are going through, both physically and emotionally.

2. **Support your healthy diet.**

This may be a difficult ask, especially if your family is used to having a lot of junk food in the home. If they are not willing to completely change their own diet, they could agree to not eat the food around you, and make sure to not leave any in the home.

3. **Give you space.**

If your family is used to you doing a lot for them, you can ask them to give you time for yourself to concentrate on the work you need to do to feel better.

Keep the Lines of Communication Open

Things are always changing, and each day will bring new triumphs and new challenges. Changing your habits is necessary but not easy. You have had years to establish those old habits, and when things feel hard, and your emotions run high, it would be so easy to run back to those old, comfortable ways.

THESE ARE THE MOMENTS WHERE YOU NEED THE MOST SUPPORT. Talk to your family daily. Let them know how you are doing. Share your wins and your worries. But most of all, tell them when you need a mood lift!

One thing you should always do is let them know just how much their help means to you. If you get through a day without resorting to eating badly, and it is because they were there to help you through it, let them know. Let them know every single time!

In the Home

Picture this:

It has been two weeks since you decided to work on changing your eating habits for the better. You have consulted a nutritionist and have come up with a meal plan that you are happy with. It provides you with plenty of tasty meal options that do not leave you starving and unhappy. It is not perfect, but it works.

It has been a long day. Your friend shared some bad news with you, you dropped a full carton of eggs on the back seat of your car (luckily, only three of them broke), and you are really, really craving a pop (or sugary soda, depending on where you are from). You have fought it all day, but it has been plaguing your brain like one of those irritating songs that get in your head.

You open the fridge to put in your nine remaining eggs, and then you see it: a big bottle of pop, right there, calling to you from the middle of the fridge. Your mouth waters and you reach for it…

What happened next did not have to happen. You had fought your craving and had made it through two entire weeks without caving. That one moment was when your family member failed you.

I know that it is hard to ask your family to change their eating habits to support you, but think of it this way:

1. Your life depends on it.

2. They will be healthier for it.

3. They love you and will miss you so much more than they will that bottle of pop.

So here is a good game plan for removing all of the junk from your home:

1. Talk to your family. Let them know how important it is, especially in the beginning, to remove all of the junk food from the house. This will ensure that your environment, at least while at home, is clear of all potential setbacks.

2. You do not have to throw out all of the food that you already have if you want to avoid waste. Finish everything that is in the house, and then do not buy any more. Replace the bad stuff with the good stuff.

3. It is that simple. No one in the family should be bringing into the house any more of the food that will tempt you.

Yes, I know that it is a challenge. But you can do it. Why? Because your life depends on it. And your family can do it. Why? Because your life depends on it.

Reach Out

Earlier, we talked briefly about what to do if you live alone, and I think we should talk a little more about it because, just in case you did not get the message earlier, your success in establishing a healthier lifestyle depends on you having the support you need. So, start by thinking about all the relatives you have on this planet. No matter where they are in the world, they are only a call, an email, or a video chat away. Reach out to them and start a conversation.

If you have not had a close relationship, simply start by reconnecting. Find out how they are. Open the line of communication. When or if you feel you have come to a place in your relationship where you can share what you are going through, start slowly.

Reach out to friends. Set up a phone call or a coffee date. If they are truly friends that have your best interest at heart, they will be there for you.

If family, relatives, and friends are not an option in your life, it is time to reach out to the broader community. Here are a few suggestions for people to turn to:

1. Like I mentioned earlier, ask your doctor for recommendations. They may think it is a good idea to talk to a therapist, or be able to give you a referral for a group program at a local hospital or community center.

2. Take a fitness class at a local community center. You could take a line dancing class or gentle yoga, or even try aquafit. The benefit to going to a regular class is that you will meet people who may become friends that you can schedule other social events with. The added bonus is that you will also be getting active!

3. If you are an older adult, many communities have centers where you can join a regular card game or attend creative arts classes.

4. Volunteer for an organization that you feel drawn too. Often, there will be other volunteers there that share your interests, who you may connect with.

5. Join an online community. Facebook often has groups that are focused on a common interest, where you can reach out and talk with others. I do not recommend that this be your only

support network, but it is a supplementary option.

6. Hire a coach. There are many coaches in the online space, who serve those who have goals they want to achieve in their life, and know they need some help.

Do whatever you can to find the support you need in achieving your health goals. When looking for support, start with your inner circle and then look to the outer circles.

Be the Support

The second part of this chapter is for the family member or friend who is your support network. Or you, if you are reading this book to learn more about your loved one's health and how you can help.

When you love someone who is struggling with their health, it can cause a lot of stress, worry, and sadness, not only for that person but for you as well. Throughout the process of learning, understanding, accepting, and growing, it is so important for you to be kind to yourself.

Keep in mind that you are helping your family member, not saving them.

Be there for them.
Listen to them.
Hold their hand.
Support their healthy lifestyle choices.

But do not do everything for them. This is actually more detrimental to their health, and to yours. As couples age, and one partner's health declines, it is common for the healthier partner to take on the role of caregiver. Did you also know that there is something called caregiver syndrome?

The role of caregiver can take its toll, and sometimes the caregiver dies before the patient, due to stress-related illness. So, when providing support:

Be there for them.
Listen to them.
Hold their hand.
Support their healthy lifestyle choices.
But set your boundaries and know when you need help too.

Don't Wait

Have you ever felt so down that you were sure that everyone around could tell how much you were hurting? Things felt so bad that you imagined that there must be a stormy cloud following you around all day. Surely, it was not just you who could see it.

Or have you ever had a friend that was the life of the party—they always seemed so happy, so put together—and once in a while, you felt a little jealous because your togetherness was not at their level? Then one day, you find out that they have taken a leave of absence from work because they are too depressed to get out of bed.

People do not always wear their emotions on the outside. Sometimes you need to be the one to ask how they are doing. I know what you might be thinking: "I have been married to my wife for 29 years; I think I know when she is feeling down."

Yes, a lot of the time you will be able to sense her change in mood or attitude before a coworker, but there are times when you cannot. That is reality! We put on a good face even for our loved ones. So, do not wait; ASK!

Make it a regular habit to ask how your loved one is doing. It can be hard to remember to do this when life gets busy, but make a routine of it. If you are morning people, sit down over breakfast and talk about how you are both doing. Just talk.

Sometimes it may be hard for your loved one to open up, especially if they are really hurting. That is okay. Let them know you will be there for them when they are ready. But again, do not wait; ASK. You are not being annoying; you are showing you care.

DO NOT WAIT; ASK!

If this is something new for your relationship, I understand. We are all different in the way that we love and the way we communicate. If you are not used to openly talking about your feelings with your partner, or your parent or sibling, it can be really hard to change that pattern. Sometimes the best thing to do is keep it simple: "How are you feeling today?" Sometimes it is nice to change it up so your loved one is not always focused on their illness. You can ask things like:

What are you looking forward to today?
What do you feel good about?
Have you discovered any new foods you like?

If you are ever stuck for something to say, all you have to do is say:

I am here to help you. I am here for you. When you are ready, let me know what you need.

Support Healthy Habits

So, you cannot have junk food in your house anymore. You like the occasional sugary drink and bag of chips. You are used to heating up a pizza for dinner on the days when cooking feels too much like work. A sweet treat before bed is something you have been doing for years. I mean, do they not leave those chocolate mints on your pillow at night in the fancy hotels? Clearly, it is okay to have a little chocolate before bed.

Now, that all has to change, and you are not sure you want it to. You have not had the same wake-up call with your health, and you know it is a good thing for everyone, but it still does not feel good. Some foods make us feel happier; that is why they are called comfort food. The great thing about comfort food is that you get to decide what makes you happy. It is all about changing your mindset and your habits.

The reality is, your loved one will not succeed, especially in the beginning, if they are surrounded by all the things they used to be able to eat and now cannot. It needs to be removed from their environment, which means it needs to be removed from yours too. In the long run, both you and I know you will feel better for it too.

The best way to lead is by example, always. That old saying, "Do as I say, not as I do," should have actually been, "Do as I do, not as I say." Our learned behaviors come more from observing than they do from taking orders. In this case, your loved one is not a child, but it is still helpful to feel the shift of energy around them. Rather than fighting the pull of old habits, they are riding the energy of new healthier habits.

Working toward a healthier lifestyle together can also bring you closer to your goal in a shorter period of time.

Success in numbers! You have the ability to be a positive agent of change, in not only your loved ones life but in your own as well.

Get excited about the change. Do some research. Try new foods. Create new healthy eating habits. Get involved! But most important of all, do not beat yourself up if you fail one day and eat something you had been trying to cut out. Be kind to yourself, enjoy the food, and then let it go. Just because you ate it once, does not mean you have to give up entirely.

KEEP GOING!

Both your life and the life of your loved one depends on it!

Take Care of You

Make time...

This is an important one! Take care of yourself too. Your life and your health are also a priority; not only in the care of your loved one but also for you.

One of the best gifts you can give yourself is time; time to do something you enjoy every single day. It is easy to get bogged down in all of the things you have to do. Create time for yourself, even if some days it is just to spend 15 minutes in the morning to catch up on the daily news.

If you have lost sight of the things that bring you joy, start by writing out a list of all the things you love to do. Ask yourself this:

1. Is there anything I used to do that I have not had time for, that I would love to try again?

2. Is there something new that I want to learn but have been putting off?

3. What are the things I can do for myself that will help me feel great about the way I look?

4. What activities help me to relax?

Once you have your list, make sure to schedule these activities into your daily schedule. If it helps, use a monthly calendar and actually write them in. Make sure to allot the amount of time you need for each, and give yourself permission to take that time. You are worth it. Your life matters.

The activities on the list are the things that keep us going in our day-to-day lives. What about the bigger things, like travel? Write out a list of places in the world you have always wanted to go but have not gotten around to going to. Or, are there places you have been that you want to go again?

Do not let diabetes stop you and your loved one from dreaming big. If you want something enough, you will start to take the necessary actions to make it happen.

Set boundaries...

Setting boundaries is not mean, and it does not mean that you are ignoring the needs of your loved one. It actually means you want to see them thrive. Saving them is not helping them; supporting them along their journey is.

For example, if they do not have the energy to do their laundry one week, and you want to help them, go for it; but do not make it a regular habit. When it is time to do laundry the next time, and you notice it is not getting done, rather than just doing it for them, ask if you could do it together.

Keep the lines of communication open. If you are starting to feel overwhelmed, let your loved one know. If they are physically unable to help around the home, it might be time to consider your options in regard to getting outside help.

The bottom line: When supporting a loved one in achieving better health and a higher quality of life, make sure you do not lose yourself in the process. Your life matters. You matter. Your loved one wants you to be happy and healthy, just as much as you want the same for them.

Enjoy Life Together

It is that simple. Enjoy life together. Enjoy each other.

Eat better.
Get active.
Enjoy each other's company.
Have fun together.
Dream bigger.

Health-Happy Lunch #2

- Stir fry mixed vegetables

- Curried chickpeas

- Small bowl of rice

- Small bowl of vegetable broth

Dessert

- 1 slice of applesauce cake

- Herbal tea or coffee

- cup of hot water

CHAPTER 6

Love Yourself

Your Life Is Worth It!

"Love yourself first and everything else falls into line. You really have to love yourself to get anything done in this world."

– Lucille Ball

6

When I sat down to brainstorm on the steps I believe you can use to take control of your diabetes and live a healthier life, one of the areas I wanted to discuss was depression. In the first five chapters, I have already addressed a lot of the ways in which we can lift our mood: good food, family, and exercise. But a low mood is not depression. Depression is bigger. The topic is much too big for one chapter in a book.

Having experienced depression in my own life, I know that the journey back to mental health is unique, but that the early warning signs are generally not. As a part of my program, I will address those signs and one of the most valuable tools for stopping depression in its tracks.

The Fork in the Road

There is always a point when you get to choose. In fact, there are many. Each and every moment of every day, you get to choose whether or not you want to feel better. Yes, it is on you. You are in fact the only person that can save yourself, because in the end, you have to be the one to decide to accept help when you need it.

So, make a choice to make your life a priority. You, your family, and your friends will thank you for it. I did start that sentence with *you* for a reason. In your life, you should always be the most important person. You are the #1 VIP. If you are not this in your own life, you will not be in anyone else's life either. Go ahead; roll out the red carpet, and put on your finest. This is your life, and it matters.

Whenever you hit that fork in the road and have to choose between making your mental health a priority or sinking deeper into a dark place, turn down the lighter path. If you can not make that choice for yourself, it is time to seek help. Let your family know. Talk to your doctor. Seeking help is choosing the path to better mental health.

Read the Signs

The early warning signs that you are experiencing depression are easy to read but not easy to ignore. Some of the symptoms you may experience are:

1. Lack of appetite

2. Not wanting to engage in daily life

3. Feeling anti-social

4. No energy

5. A strong desire to stay in bed all day

In the beginning, you may be able to take on these warning signs by doing some of the things we already talked about, like eating well, seeking the support of your family, getting active, and taking care of your hygiene. But if it progresses, you will need to seek help.

Some of the signs that you are depressed:

1. Suicidal thoughts

2. Sleeping all the time

3. Not bathing

4. Cancelling all social plans

5. Lack of ability to experience joy in activities you used to love

If you cannot help yourself, get help. If you notice these behaviors in a loved one, help them get help.

The most important message you will read in this chapter:

You are worth it. Your life matters!

Stop Depression in Its Tracks

The most powerful tool you can add to your toolbox in building stronger mental health is love for yourself. I know, I know; it is cliché, but it is true. Strong mental health begins with loving yourself. When you love yourself, you realize that **YOU ARE WORTH IT** and **YOUR LIFE MATTERS.**

Loving yourself is always the first step, but it is much easier said than done. We have so many complicated emotions when it comes to loving ourselves, especially if we have been diagnosed with a disease that makes us feel like we can not do all of the things we used to.

As we age, and the years chip away at the things we used to do and took pride in, it can be a challenge to maintain a sense of self-worth. A lack of self-worth can serve to diminish the love we feel for ourselves. So for me, when I feel myself slipping into depression, the first thing I want to do is strengthen my love for myself by recognizing my own self-worth.

One of the first things I want you to do is get a sheet of paper or a journal and a pen. Do not wait; get it now.

Are you still reading?
I was serious.
Go!
I will be here when you get back.
Got it?

Good. Let's write! This may feel silly or weird, or make you angry or annoyed, or make you feel like you have nothing to say. All of these things are normal. Self-reflection is not something that a majority of this world does on a daily basis. It may take you out of your comfort zone. That is exactly where you want to go.

Begin by writing out 7 things you love about yourself, with *I am* statements.

Here are mine:

1. I am loving.
2. I am compassionate.
3. I am open to new adventures.
4. I am intelligent.
5. I am willing to try new things.
6. I am kind to myself and others.
7. I am interested in making the world a healthier place.

You will notice that my responses are very general. They could apply to anyone. Now I want to go a bit deeper and make them more specific to my life, by proving my *I am* statements right. Take each statement and ask yourself when in your life you have proven it to be correct. For example:

1. I am loving.
Every day, I show myself love by eating well and participating in activities that I love, like taking

a dance class. I show my family love by cooking healthy meals for them and spending quality time with them. I show the world love by reducing waste whenever possible, and trying to get better at it every day.

2. I am compassionate.
I check in on my close friends to make sure they are okay when they are going through a rough time. I do not judge others when they need to vent about the challenges they are facing. I always try to find a way to inspire them to feel better. For example, when my sister was with me, I inspired her to get active and lead a healthier life, by doing it with her.

3. I am open to new adventures.
I love exploring the world around me. Whether it is a walking path in a neighboring town or a farmer's market across the ocean, I am always ready to get out there and see what this world has to offer.

4. I am intelligent.
I have always been smart enough to tackle any job that I wanted, even if I was not skilled at it right away. When I do not understand something, I find the resources I need in order to help me learn.

5. I am willing to try new things.

If you would have told me 10 years ago that I would be an author one day, I would have stared at you in disbelief. But here I am today; you are reading this book because I decided to take a leap of faith, trust in myself, and try something new.

6. I am kind to myself and others.

There are times when it is hard to be kind, especially if someone is treating me badly or when I am annoyed with a perceived shortcoming in myself. But for the most part, I choose kindness. I have the patience to sit back and wait for the emotions to pass, so that I can be the person I know I am.

7. I am interested in making the world a healthier place.

After witnessing what my sister went through, and learning all that I had to learn to help her, I now feel like I cannot keep this knowledge in. It needs to be shared, and even if one person achieves a better quality of life, then I have succeeded.

Sometimes when we write these statements, we think we believe them, but in fact we do not. Your subconscious mind is working away behind the scenes to prove you wrong. It will dig up any memory it can get its little neurons on to challenge your belief in your new I AM statements. Why? I am not 100% sure really, but I feel it myself.

Like when I say *I am kind to myself,* that little voice in the back of my head responds with: *hmmm… you must be forgetting that just this morning you called yourself stupid for putting your hair brush back in the wrong spot, and then forgetting where that spot was.*

Or when I say *I am intelligent,* that annoying little voice jumps in loud and clear with: *but don't you remember how hard you had to work to understand any complex math problems in high school. And just the other day…*

My own personal ideal on why we find it easier to beat ourselves up rather than build ourselves up, is simple: We have been beating ourselves up for years. We are used to doing it. Change is hard. Change takes work. Change, especially with thought patterns, takes repetition. A few ways that you can strengthen your own belief in these *I am* statements is to read them every morning when you get up, write them over and over again, and add proof each day as things happen.

You Are Your Light

"Is life worth living? It all depends on the liver."

– William James

Your life is 100%, without a doubt, worth living, because YOU are worth it, and YOUR life matters. I could say that over and over and over again. We all need to hear it, as often as possible. It is so easy to forget. It is so easy to get lost in all of the things that are going wrong. It is so easy to drown in your own negative beliefs about yourself. Whenever you feel yourself slipping, always come back to this:

You are worth it. Your life matters!

You are the one and only person in this world that needs to believe that. It is true. Of course, you want others to see you, to understand you, to support you, to need you, and to love you, but in the end, the one person who needs to believe that your life matters is you.

How can you be the light you need to be for yourself?

This begins with the love we just talked about. When you love yourself, you know you are worth it. It is something that you understand intrinsically. Of course, you are worth it; why wouldn't you be? Obviously, your life matters; how could it not?

Over time, if you have slowly stopped loving yourself and are stuck in self-limiting beliefs, it is hard to remember that your life matters. Some of these self-limiting beliefs come from years of negative thought patterns and behaviors, while some may have been brought on by your declining health and your diabetes diagnosis. You may be thinking things like:

- I used to be useful, but now I can barely do anything.

- No one needs me.

- I am a burden to my family, and it will only get worse.

- I can't beat this. What's the point in trying?

- It is too late for me to try anything new.

- I let things go too far to fix them now.

- I am lazy.

These thoughts only serve to reduce your worth in your own eyes. They are in fact useless. They have no purpose other than to bring you down and keep you there. The best thing to do when faced with these limiting beliefs is fight fire with fire; meaning take a negative belief and knock it down with a positive belief.

To show you what I mean, I am going to take my self-limiting beliefs from above and fight them with a positive, self-affirming belief:

- I used to be useful, but now I can barely do anything. – **I am useful in so many ways.**

- No one needs me. – **The world needs me and my positive energy.**

- I am a burden to my family, and it will only get worse. – **I am an important part of my family and will never be a burden to them.**

- I can't beat this. What's the point in trying? – **I can do anything I set my mind to, and my life is worth fighting for.**

- It is too late for me to try anything new. – **Learning new things gets me excited for each day. It is never too late to try something different.**

- I let things go too far to fix them now. – **Right now is the exact right time to make the change I need in order to feel better.**

- I am lazy. – **I am motivated to make my health a priority, and I am ready to do the work.**

Your thoughts ultimately control your actions and reactions. Strengthen your brain muscle, and you will be able to deal with all of the challenges life throws your way, even diabetes. You can improve your quality of life by controlling your thoughts. You might be thinking: *How the heck does that work?* Easy! Your thoughts become your reality. If you think something enough, you come to believe it, and if you come to believe it, then your decisions are affected by that belief.

Imagine that a good friend calls you up one day and says:

"You are never going to believe this! I have been calling into this radio for years, trying to win one of their trips. The most I ever got was a mug with their name on it, along with a promotional pen that lasted for about a week. Well, last week, that changed. I won an all-inclusive cruise on the Danube. Flights and everything. For two! Wanna come?"

You think about it for a minute. You are not feeling great. It was difficult to get in the shower the other day, and you had not kept to your walking schedule the last couple of weeks. You knew you were going downhill and did not feel like there was any chance that it was going to get better any time soon. The thought of saying no made you really sad and angry with yourself, but ultimately you did not want to ruin your friend's trip.

"Congratulations, that is so amazing! But I am just not feeling up to it. I will just slow you down. How about Meaghan? Have you checked with her?"

"NO! I want you to come. I thought of you first because you are my best friend, and even if we do move a little slower, who cares? We always have fun together! You're my first choice; pleeeeeeeease..."

One of two things could happen next:

1. *You are unable to really hear how much your friend wants you to go because your negative thoughts get in the way of you hearing the truth. All you hear is that you will be a burden and add an element of worry to the trip, which would not be there if a more mobile friend went along. This way of thinking only brings on more negative thoughts, allowing you to devalue yourself and your life even further.*

2. *You snap out of it and realize what an amazing opportunity this is. A free cruise on the Danube. That offer was not going to come back your way anytime soon. Not only that, but you can remember having fun. You love to travel, and you embrace all that exploring new places has to offer. And last but not least, this is your best friend. You know that you would never, ever be considered a burden to her. So you say "yes," and you do not allow yourself to miss out on the trip of a lifetime.*

Your thoughts inform your actions, and ultimately become your life. If you feel yourself slipping into negativity, take control. You are your light. You have all that you need within yourself to live a life that you are excited about each day.

Take a Breather

One of the best things you can do for yourself when you feel you are slipping into a negative thought process is to breathe. For example, with the example above, if you find yourself still feeling like you have to say *no*, when you really, really want to go, ask for some time. Let your friend know that you are so grateful she chose you to share this amazing gift, but that you need a day to think about it.

Take some time to yourself and literally just breathe. It is simple. Find yourself a quiet spot in the house, and ask anyone who is at home at the time to not disturb you for five minutes. Make yourself comfortable and close your eyes. Focus on breathing deeply. You want to think about sending the oxygen way down into your diaphragm, which are the muscles that separate your chest from your abdomen. Place your hands there while you breathe, and feel the muscles expand and contract as you inhale and exhale.

For five minutes, just sit and breathe. This will help center you and allow you to start your thought process from a fresh place with a positive perspective.

Your Life Matters

Oh, have I already told you that your life matters?
I have. Right! I have, a few times now.

I actually know that, but it is a big, important fact. It is a fact. It is not debatable. It is non-negotiable. It is a fact.

This can be hard to remember, especially when going through tough times. You start to feel like maybe your life does not actually matter. You start to think small, and so you start to feel small. You are sliding down a very slippery slope!

"Your life matters" is an easy thing to say, but if you are used to putting everyone and everything ahead of yourself, it can be a hard thing to act on. It all comes back to your beliefs. I am normally not one to work with this many affirmations in one chapter, but when it comes to changing your limiting self-beliefs, they work. You cannot just write it out once and expect your brain to believe it. Make writing out these affirmations a daily practice, or put them up where you can read them every day. But then you need to act on those affirmations. That last point is key.

The affirmations:

1. My life is important.

2. I am the master of my life.

3. I get to choose.

4. I am more than enough.

The actions:

1. **My life is important.** – Make healthy food choices because you value your life and therefore your body.

2. **I am the master of my life.** – Take control of your day and do things that make you happy.

3. **I get to choose.** – Take the trip! There is always a way. The choice is yours.

4. **I am more than enough.** – Stop beating yourself up for not being able to do everything you used to. You are more than enough. Give yourself credit for all the good that you are and do.

Make a choice to reframe your self-limiting beliefs; take action on the reframing, and then watch your quality of life as well as your mood get better.

Show Yourself Some Love

One of the best ways to convince yourself and believe that you are worthy and your life is important, is to show yourself some love. This step is fun, and there are a few ways you can make yourself feel authentically loved by you.

The first one is… can you guess it! Eat quality food. Give your body the best, and it will feel the love—no words necessary with this one.

The second way is to congratulate yourself for all the good you do. You do not have to jump into a raging current to save a terrified puppy from drowning. You do not have to run a marathon. You do not even have to come up with a lifesaving cure for cancer. I mean, if you could do any of these things, and the opportunity presented itself, then yep, you deserve some serious celebration. But really, why not give yourself the recognition you deserve for pushing your way out of bed on those days when your body aches everywhere, and it would be so much easier to stay all tucked in? Why not give yourself credit for reaching out to a friend in need and taking them out for coffee? You do a whole bunch of good in the world, but you do not see it because you are not open to it. My challenge for you is to recognize all the good you do.

The third, and in my opinion, most fun way to show just how much I love myself, is by doing something I love every single day. I go for a long walk in the sunshine. I sit down for half an hour by myself, to read. I learn a new recipe. I meet my friends for dinner. Make a commitment to yourself to include activities that you love in your life, every single day. Create a schedule and put it up on your fridge, or add the activities as appointments in your phone.

Give yourself the gift of better health, more mobility, and fun activities to get you excited about the day.

Visualization Exercise

There is no doubt that you will get discouraged some days. You are working toward living healthier, and you have done a lot of work to establish better habits, and yet your numbers are not getting any lower. You feel lethargic some days, and it feels easier to just give up rather than go on.

That is your limiting beliefs kicking back to your old habits. Do not let them! Focus on the process and not the end goal. Congratulate yourself, show yourself some love, and always, always, always remind yourself that you are worth it.

I wanted to end this chapter by sharing with you a visualization to help you get through some of the harder days.

Begin your visualization with the breath exercise I shared earlier in the chapter. Now imagine yourself sitting in your favorite place in the whole, entire world. Is it a beach? Is it a mountain top? Is it your family cottage? Is it your own backyard?

Wherever this place is, you feel safe, comfortable, and happy. You feel healthy. In this place, you can do anything—you can fly, you can leap, you can twirl, you can run. Your thoughts feel clear, and your body is full of energy. Stand up, and start running, flying, leaping, or twirling.

When you are ready, imagine yourself falling back onto a soft, comfortable surface. You are happy. You feel accomplished. You feel healthy.

When you are ready, open your eyes.

Health-Happy Treat

Turkey and Chickpea Curry

Ingredients:

2 tbsp. vegetable oil
1 lb. turkey breast, sliced into steaks
1 onion, thinly sliced
2 tbsp. curry, mixed with 1/4 cup water or 1/4 cup curry paste
1 28-oz. can chickpeas, drained
1 cup tomato puree
1 sprig of fresh curry leaves
1/4 cup chopped fresh coriander leaves
2 cups baby spinach

Method:

Place 1 tbsp. oil in pan over medium heat; brown turkey on all sides, for about 3–4 minutes, and just cook through. Transfer to a bowl.

Heat remaining oil in a pan over medium heat. Add onion, stirring for 10 minutes or until softened; add curry, stirring for about 1–2 minutes. Add chickpeas and stir to coat; add tomato puree and 1 cup cold water, and season with salt and pepper. Bring to a boil. Reduce heat to medium-low. Add curry leaves, Simmer for 15 minutes or until sauce is thickened. Return turkey to sauce. Stir to combine. Cook for 5 minutes or until heated through.

Stir in 2 cups of baby spinach.

Serve over steamed Tilda basmati rice and steamed broccoli.

Enjoy with a glass of wine.

CHAPTER 7

Get Social

It's Good for You!

*"Surround yourself with only
people who are going
to lift you higher."*

– Oprah Winfrey

7

Talk About It

One of the best things you can do for yourself is to talk about what you are going through. As we have already discussed earlier in this chapter, talk about it with family and with friends. Find a supportive ear in those who love you.

That being said, one of the best things you can do for yourself is talk about it with someone that is going through it. They will understand what you are going through on a level that others will not, because they have been there. They have experienced physical pain. They know what it feels like to have to change their diet. They understand what it feels like when they fail to stay on their diet. Basically, their empathy comes from a place of understanding.

Connect with your doctor to see if there is a diabetes support group at your local community center or outreach program. You can also search Meetup groups in your area. There are so many benefits to talking about diabetes with others:

1. You feel less alone.

2. You feel supported in your journey by others who are going through it.

3. You are getting out of the house and interacting with others.

4. Meeting others who are going through similar challenges, normalizes your condition.

5. You learn tips and tricks from others, which will help you stick to your healthy lifestyle.

6. You have the opportunity to support someone else. This reminds you that you have value to share, which can give you your power back.

There are so many benefits to talking about diabetes with others who have it. Often, especially in Western culture, we look to the more physical remedies to heal our illness: like eating well, taking medications, getting enough sleep, and exercising. If these things become overwhelming, things like talking about diabetes can improve mental health.

TALK ABOUT IT!

How Does Being Social Boost Your Health?

In a way, getting out there and being with others is actually just like taking a pill. Being with others is known to lower your stress, which has huge positive effects on how your body feels physically. Stress causes the body to feel heavy and lethargic. When you allow stress to live in the body, it can cause a myriad of health problems. High stress levels can harm the well-being of every system in the body. So, get out there, and get social to relieve some of that stress.

Getting social adds years to your life! It is true. According to a study conducted at Brigham-Young University, loneliness and isolation can be worse for you than obesity. Do not get me wrong here; I am not saying you should let go of your diet in favor of socializing. What I am saying is that you are doing yourself harm by not getting out there and being with people.[6]

There have been studies that show how being social also helps you to establish and successfully maintain healthier habits. Specifically, studies that have come out of Maastricht Medical Centre, in the Netherlands, showed that people who were socially active had decreased risks of developing type 2 diabetes.[7]

One last study for you: Researchers at Duke University Medical Centre found that those with serious medical conditions, who have strong social connections, were more likely to live longer.[8]

---

6 https://www.nextavenue.org/6-health-benefits-being-social/

7 https://www.medicalnewstoday.com/articles/321019#Social-context-determines-healthful-habits

8 https://www.nytimes.com/2017/06/12/well/live/having-friends-is-good-for-you.html

Are you convinced yet? Healing, growing, and beating your diabetes diagnosis is not about the diabetes itself. It is about you. It is about you as a person. Your life is more than your illness, so when you treat the entirety of who you are, rather than just focusing on treating the disease, you are missing out on a large opportunity for healing. Healing your whole self requires that you get out there and be with people.

Look Up

One of the biggest misconceptions is that it is hard to meet new friends as you get older. This is absolutely not true! The one stopping you from meeting new friends is YOU! Yep, there are a ton of people out there in the world who would love to know you. You are letting this one limiting belief hold you back from meeting new, amazing people who will enrich your life. Not only that, but you are preventing them from having their life enriched by you.

Why?

Why are you holding yourself back from happiness? New friends are so beneficial to every stage of life. It's always amazing to me that people stop trying to make new friends. When you were in school, you probably chose your friends based on your age, who was in your class, or who lived the closest to you on the street you grew up on.

As you got older, you might have met people in college or through your career. But life got busy. You might have had kids. You might have had ailing parents to take care of. You might have had an incredibly demanding career. Time with friends could have become less and less.

Now that you are older, you have more time. Wouldn't it be nice to make new friends? New friends are amazing for our health and happiness, for so many reasons:

1. New friends introduce you to new activities. New activities are amazing for the brain!

2. New friends see things in you that your old friends might not see. They remind you of all the good you have in you.

3. New friends shake you out of your comfort zone.

4. New friends give you the opportunity to expand your community.

5. New friends have different stories and memories to share.

6. New friends expand your world.

How do you meet new friends?

The answer to this is really simple: LOOK UP.

How often do you find yourself going about your usual errands or daily routines with your head down? Your day is a checklist, and you are focused on achieving all that you have set out to achieve. This is no way to live. It is certainly not helping you feel healthier and happier. You are not a robot!

LOOK UP, and make eye contact with people. Talk to the man sitting next to you on the bus; make small talk with the woman waiting for her prescription at the drugstore. You may not make a lasting friendship by engaging in a bit of conversation while out in public, but you never know unless you try.

If you have joined a community center, find out if there is a group that plays cards. Even if you do not play cards, give it a go. It is a great place to chat with new people.

If you volunteer for a charity organization, connect with the other volunteers. Do not just put in your time and leave. Say yes to attending any extra social functions they might organize for the volunteers. Is it a hospital or a retirement home you work for? Sometimes there are opportunities to assist with group outings. Jump on those opportunities, and talk to everyone.

Another big limiting belief is that young people are not interested in talking to older people. Why not just reach out and talk to someone, regardless of these gaps. You never know, you both might have something in common! Before you stop yourself from reaching out to someone because you have made an assumption that they will not want to talk to you, remember that everyone needs friends, and you are not the only one who might be feeling lonely.

All social interaction is a two-way street. It is a win-win! Everyone benefits. You both have made each other's day better by connecting. The bottom line is: LOOK UP and reach out. There are so many people in this world, and a lot of them would love to talk to you.

Keep Your Curiosity Alive

Did you know that one of the best things you can do for your brain is to learn new things? It turns out that this is also great for your health. Having purpose, and feeling useful, gives your life meaning, and when your life has meaning, you are willing to fight for yourself.

One of the things I do to keep my curiosity alive is to attend networking events. At these events, I learn a ton of new things and meet the most interesting people. If it were not for one of these events, I would not be writing this book. Did you read that? I started writing a book, one in which I have the opportunity to share my message with others, all because I challenged myself to get out there and try something new.

Have you ever thought of writing a book? What has stopped you? Have you ever thought of starting your own business? Yes, now! It does not matter how old you are; it is never too late to fulfill your heart's desire or your soul's calling.

What on earth does this have to do with the benefits of being social, you ask?

Well, that is easy! When you meet new people, you give yourself the opportunity to be influenced by new ways of thinking and new ways of doing. If you surround yourself with those who are all doom and gloom, then your life will be doom and gloom. If you surround yourself with interesting people who always have new ideas and are ready to give them a try, you will be inspired to do the same.

Keep your mind curious and open to the new and exciting things that new connections have to offer. There are many health benefits to this! Going back to this idea of treating you as a person rather than your diagnosis:

1. You are giving yourself the power to dream.
2. You are living life rather than focusing on your health.
3. You are raising your energy and mood by actively designing your days.
4. You are connecting with others in a meaningful way.

Social engagement and interaction can be about having a fun conversation with the ladies over lunch, an interesting debate with your book club over a controversial topic, or inspiring others as well as yourself to keep striving for more.

Look for opportunities to network with like-minded folks, in the newspaper, online, at your local community center, or at a lifelong learning program at your community college. There are many opportunities for you to continue to pursue your dreams, as long as you are willing to look.

Get Social Over Tea

In that last section, I talked a lot about getting out there and engaging in social activities that inspire you to keep striving for your dreams, no matter what stage of life you are in. For this section, I want to look at getting inspired to create fun and different types of social activities, to inspire you to stay social.

One of the fun ones that I have done with my friends is to get a group going where we have afternoon tea at each other's homes. It is easy to organize and really fun. Smaller groups for this type of event work really well— 4 or 5 at the most. You want it to be easy to organize so that it does not become an overwhelming task.

Create a schedule, like every second Tuesday of the month, and then assign who will host each tea. You can ask everyone to bring a small treat to share with the group. You can keep it simple or go more elaborate. Maybe once every few months, you could make it a fun dress-up event, where everyone wears fun fascinators.

Get Competitive

Have you ever held a game night? They are so fun! You can organize this type of recurring event exactly like the afternoon tea. Get a group of people together, create a schedule, and rotate the hosts. Everyone brings a snack to share. To keep it fun and exciting, always introduce new games into the mix.

Another great way to get competitive while being social is to join a bowling league. They usually meet once a week, and it is the type of game where you can still talk to others while playing. If you have not tried it, I highly recommend it.

Take a Day Trip

When was the last time you explored your city, town, or surrounding area, like a tourist? This is not only incredibly fun, but also a great way to connect with others. You can either go solo or join a group. If you do go solo, remember to look up and talk to people. It is an adventure! If you see the magic in every day, you will find yourself experiencing it.

If you would rather go with a group, check out your local senior's center or community center. They often organize day trips that provide transportation and an opportunity to connect with those you are traveling with.

Another great way to explore the city with people is to research Meetup groups in your area. There might be some that regularly go exploring the area together. Sometimes you can even find something like a photography walk, where you can join others in viewing your city through the creative eye of a camera lens.

Some of the places you can explore are:

1. Museums
2. Art galleries
3. Historic sites
4. Conservation areas
5. Wildlife sanctuaries
6. Amusement parks
7. Casinos
8. Art festivals
9. Seasonal festivals
10. Farmer's markets

If your city is a tourist destination, why not take a bike tour or hop on one of those tour buses that guide you through the city. Sometimes there are things like winery tours, pub tours, and even haunted house tours. Take an adventure. It can never hurt. You never know who you will meet or what you will learn!

Get Outta Town

How long has it been since you took a vacation? Now, how long has it been since you joined a tour group? For some of you reading this, I imagine the answer would be "never." If you need some help finding a trip that is best suited to your needs, why not chat with a travel agent. They can tell you all about what is available to you, depending on the criteria you give them.

How far do you want to go? How long do you want to go for? How much money do you want to spend? How much of the trip do you want to spend on a guided group tour?

You could take a weekend trip to a city in another province, or you could take a riverboat cruise down the Danube.

Do not let your fear and worries stop you. Keep dreaming. Keep doing. When you open yourself up to possibilities, especially ones that involve new friends, you allow yourself to keep living. When you allow yourself to keep living, you prove to yourself that you are worth it and your health matters.

Hold Yourself Accountable

Place importance on being socially active. It might be the last thing on your list when you are focused on getting all of life's to-do's done while changing your diet, exercising, and really focusing on your health, but as you have seen, it is just as important.

Do your research and find new activities in your area. Challenge yourself to step outside your comfort zone and join a new group alone. It is always fun to travel with friends, but sometimes if you want to meet new people, it is good to get out there by yourself. You are more likely to talk to someone new when you do not have your friend there to keep you company.

Create a schedule. Add at least one new event to it once a month. Yes, once a month. Try out a workshop, or a networking event, or go on a bus tour.

Write out your big dreams. Where in the world do you want to go? What in the world do you still want to do? Create an action plan to realize these dreams. Do not just talk about them; make them happen.

Just Get Social

I wanted to bring this chapter to a close by providing a quick recap, because I think that there are some really important points here that could help you achieve your health goals. I also feel that they get pushed in priority, behind some of the more serious tasks, when I think that getting social should hold the same weight.

Here are the facts:

1. Talking about your diabetes diagnosis with others who are going through it, gives you a much needed support network of people who can help you navigate your health journey.

2. Stress causes all of the systems in your body to break down. Staying socially engaged relieves stress and adds years to your life.

3. You can make new friends at any age. All you need to do is look up and be open to talking to a friendly stranger.

4. New friends open you up to new and potentially interesting experiences.

5. Stay curious! Head to networking events to meet new people and get inspired to do new things, like write a book or start a side business.

This is amazing for giving you purpose and direction.

6. Give yourself the gift of adventure, in your own city or abroad. Join new friends and old, in exploring the world.

7. Get social; YOUR LIFE DEPENDS ON IT!

Health-Happy Packable Lunch

- 1 cream of asparagus soup {insulated thermos food jar}

- 1 pita pocket stuffed with jerk chicken and vegetables Small container of mixed fruit

- 1 slice of egg-free, no-sugar banana bread {nice treat} Hot water {insulated thermos}

- 1 bottle of water

Enjoy!!!

CHAPTER 8

Stay Healthy

Keep an Eye on Your Health
Through Self-Monitoring

"Keeping your body healthy is an expression of gratitude to the whole cosmos—the trees, the clouds, everything."

– Thich Nhat Hanh

8

You have worked hard to change your habits. You have begun eating better. You have worked on your hygiene. You have gotten more social. You have begun to be more physically active.

YOU HAVE DONE AN AMAZING JOB!

Give yourself the credit you deserve. Changing your life takes courage, and it takes work. You are doing it. Keep going. If you are reading this and thinking that you have not made the progress you thought you would by now, STOP! You are doing amazing.

Pat yourself on the back.

Happy dance around your kitchen.

Shout it out from the rooftops!

One of the most effective ways for you to maintain the healthy lifestyle you have begun to create for yourself, is to give yourself credit for the work you are doing, and reward yourself. How are you rewarding yourself for a job well done? Create a list of healthy rewards that make you happy, like an extra half hour of reading without interruption in the evening, or a night out to see a movie of your choosing. Make sure your rewards are things that are healthy and bring you joy. Rewards are so important.

If you are only beating yourself up, there is no way you will succeed in the long run. So make sure you reward yourself for your work! Take note of the last part of that sentence: Reward yourself for THE WORK.

Why did I want you to take note of that key element? Because as you continue to monitor your health and your progress, you may not always see positive results. This is OKAY! Keep going. Do not give up!

Remember: REWARD YOURSELF FOR THE WORK, NOT THE OUTCOME

What to Monitor

There are a few things you will want to monitor specifically. What are they?

1. Your glucose levels

2. Your blood pressure

3. Your weight

4. Your water intake

5. Your mood

Glucose Levels

Monitoring your levels daily is extremely important for keeping your diabetes under control. With high or low levels of blood sugar, serious complications can develop.

With **hyperglycemia**, you have high levels of glucose in your blood. Some of the complications you can experience are:

1. Heart disease or heart attack

2. Stroke

3. Kidney damage

4. Nerve damage

5. Eye damage

6. Skin problems[9]

If your blood sugar is high, you can bring it down by cutting carbs and starchy foods (like white potatoes and rice), and reducing your sugar intake. You can replace these with foods that have a lower glycemic index.

If you want a more detailed list of foods based on their glycemic index, there are many resources available online. But for now, here are a few examples, provided

---

9 https://www.webmd.com/diabetes/uncontrolled-blood-sugar-risks

by the American Diabetes Association, of low, medium, or high GI foods:

Low GI foods (55 or less)

- 100% stone-ground whole wheat or pumpernickel bread

- Oatmeal (rolled or steel-cut), oat bran, muesli

- Pasta, converted rice, barley, bulgur

- Sweet potato, corn, yam, lima/butter beans, peas, legumes, and lentils

- Most fruits and non-starchy vegetables

Medium GI (56–69)

- Whole wheat, rye, and pita bread

- Quick oats

- Brown, wild, or basmati rice; couscous

High GI (70 or more)

- White bread or bagel

- Corn flakes, puffed rice, bran flakes, instant oatmeal

- Short-grain white rice, rice pasta, macaroni and cheese from mix

- Russet potato, pumpkin

- Pretzels, rice cakes, popcorn, saltine crackers

- Melons and pineapple[10]

With **hypoglycemia**, your blood sugar level is too low. This can be a very dangerous condition and requires medical attention immediately if the following symptoms are severe:

1. Rapid heartbeat

2. Sudden mood changes

3. Sudden nervousness

4. Unexplained fatigue

5. Pale skin

6. Headache

7. Hunger

8. Shaking

9. Dizziness

10. Sweating

---

10 https://www.diabetes.org/glycemic-index-and-diabetes

11. Difficulty sleeping

12. Skin tingling

13. Trouble thinking clearly or concentrating

14. Loss of consciousness, seizure, coma[11]

If you are experiencing these symptoms at a mild to moderate level, eat 15 grams of easily digestible carbohydrates. Some examples are:

1. Half a cup of juice or regular soda

2. 1 tablespoon of honey

3. 4 or 5 saltine crackers

4. 3 or 4 pieces of hard candy or glucose tablets

5. 1 tablespoon of sugar

Often, when people are first diagnosed with diabetes, improving their health is a top priority, so they remember to monitor their glucose levels every day. Does this sound familiar? But then as time goes on, the monitoring may get forgotten one day, and then another. Things become more relaxed. Does this still sound like you?

This is your wake-up call: MONITOR YOUR GLUCOSE LEVELS EVERY SINGLE DAY! Your life does depend

---

11 https://www.healthline.com/health/hypoglycemia#symptoms

on this. Here are a few handy tips to help you stay on top of it:

1. Figure out the best time of day for you to test, and stay consistent.

2. Set an alarm that reminds you to test.

3. Keep the testing tools handy.

4. Keep a results journal and pen with your testing kit.

5. Do not worry if you do forget one day; pick it right back up the next day.

See your doctor regularly!

One of the best ways to keep on top of your monitoring is to keep regular appointments with your doctor. Your doctor will let you know how often to come, but as a rule of thumb, I think at least once every three months is good if you are managing. At these appointments, be sure to share your daily test results with your doctor, and also make sure to have your blood tested there as well.

Blood Pressure

Often, people with type 2 diabetes will have high blood pressure, and this is why you need to remain vigilant.

High blood pressure, or hypertension, can lead to many complications, but there are ways that you can help to lower your blood pressure. Here are 10 ways according to the Mayo clinic:

1. Lose extra pounds and watch your waistline.

2. Exercise regularly.

3. Eat a healthy diet.

4. Reduce sodium in your diet.

5. Limit the amount of alcohol you drink.

6. Quit smoking.

7. Cut back on caffeine.

8. Reduce your stress.

9. Monitor your blood pressure at home, and see your doctor regularly.

10. Get support.[12]

Amazing! You are already doing many of these things the Mayo Clinic is suggesting. Now all you have to do is get yourself a home monitoring kit if you do not have one already. They range anywhere in cost from approximately thirty dollars to one-hundred and thirty

---

12 https://www.mayoclinic.org/diseases-conditions/high-blood-pressure/in-depth/high-blood-pressure/art-20046974

dollars, but they are worth it. You can even keep it handy with your glucose level kit and do it all at the same time, recording your results in the same journal.

Weight

We have already talked about this one, so I will not talk about it much more. Remember not to weigh yourself every day. There are normal fluctuations that occur that may leave you feeling like you have not made any progress. Again, do not let the numbers get you down, but rather use them as a guide. If your current dietary plan is not seeing success, why not seek some help. You could always meet with a nutritionist and have them build a plan for you. You could continue to work with them to monitor your results and adjust your plan as needed.

If you are serious about your health and achieving results, you have to seek the help you need. You cannot expect yourself to know everything right away. If you put too much pressure on yourself, you are setting yourself up to fail. Give yourself a chance, be kind to yourself, and get help!

Water

One of the absolute best things you can do for yourself is to drink water. If you drink enough water, it also has the ability to eliminate extra glucose from your body, through urine. The Institute of Medicine recommends that men drink about 13 cups per day, and women about 9 cups.[13]

Plain water, although refreshing on a hot day, can get boring. Add a little flavor to your water with some lemon or mint, to make it more appealing.

Mood

I have also talked about this a lot, but it is important. If your mood starts to dip, keep on top of it, because if you let it go too low, it will get harder to bring yourself back up. A low mood will stop you from having the motivation you need to keep the healthy lifestyle you have worked so hard to create.

When you are feeling mentally healthy, it is only natural for you to want to also take care of your physical health. So make sure to monitor your mental health as well. The easiest way to do this is by observing your own behaviors. Ask yourself these few simple questions:

1. Do I find it hard to get up in the morning?

2. Have I been cancelling my social plans because I feel too low to be around people?

---

13 https://www.healthline.com/health/diabetes/drinks-for-diabetics#best-drinks

3. Am I taking care of my hygiene?

4. Am I excited about life?

If you want, a good practice is to also add these questions in your monitoring journal. Observe your behaviors at least once a week, or even once every two weeks, whatever works for you. When your mood is consistently dipping, seek help immediately. Here are some things you can do:

1. Consult your doctor.

2. Get a referral for a therapist.

3. Talk to your family.

4. Join a support group.

Get the help you need so that you can continue to thrive!

Conclusion

Monitoring may seem like an overwhelming task, but it is really not at all. You can chunk your glucose, blood pressure, weight, and mood monitoring together. Create a weekly schedule telling you on which days you need to do what. For example:

Monday
Glucose
Blood pressure

Tuesday
Glucose
Blood pressure

Wednesday
Glucose
Blood pressure
Weight

Thursday
Glucose
Blood pressure

Friday
Glucose
Blood pressure
Mood

Saturday
Glucose
Blood pressure

Sunday
Glucose
Blood pressure

It is just like brushing your teeth. Get up in the morning, brush your teeth, monitor your health, and then move on with your day!

Health-Happy Dinner

Mashed Plantains

2 medium green plantains
2 cups water
2 tbsp. butter or olive oil

Method:

Place water in a saucepan and bring to a boil.
Peel and cut up plantains.
Add plantains to the saucepan, and cook until tender.
Remove from the stove, drain, and mash with potato masher.
Add butter, and season to taste if necessary, with a pinch of salt.
Serves two.
Enjoy.

Stovetop Steamed Black Cod

2 slices of black cod
1 medium yellow onion, chopped
2 cloves garlic, diced
1 small roma tomato, diced
1 tbsp. sesame oil
Couple pinches of kosher salt
Couple pinches of black pepper
Pinch of ground thyme

Method:

Clean and dry black cod, and set aside.

Heat oil in a frying pan.

Sauté onion, garlic, and tomato, for about 2 minutes.

Add fish to pan; season with salt, black pepper, and ground thyme.

Cover and cook for about 12 minutes until flakey. Do not overcook.

Baste fish with sauce during cooking.

Remove from heat and let sit for 3 minutes.

Serve over mashed plantain.

Serves 2.

Enjoy!!!!!!

CHAPTER 9

Make It Easy

Give Yourself the Tools You Need

"Life is what you make of it. You can make it easy on yourself or you can make it hard."

– Deep Roy

9

Did you know that life can be easy? Did you also know that oftentimes it is you who is making it hard on yourself? I know that this is a difficult truth to hear, but it is true. Think about a task in your life right now that you have to do every day. Now, ask yourself: "Have I done everything I can to make this as easy as it can be?"

A lot of the time, we do things the same way we have always done them. It is human nature to resist change. It is human nature to want to stick to the way of doing things that we understand. Think about any major change to technology that has occurred in your lifetime, especially in your adult years.

One of the things that was a huge change in my life, outside of the development of the internet, was the introduction of cellphones into our lives. I know that there is a whole generation of people, and there will be many more to come, who don't even know what life was like without them. When they first came out, there was a whole generation of people who could not believe they would replace landlines. In fact, I know people who still have landlines because they find them easier to use than cell phones.

The reality is, cell phones do make things far more convenient and often easier, as we can reach our loved ones at any time. They are also always on us, so if we have an emergency, help is always at our fingertips. That being said, why is it so hard for people to let go of using the landline? Because it is familiar. For many people, they had used a landline for decades. It is what they know.

Getting used to a new way of doing things takes work in the beginning. It's easy to think, "Oh, I will just do this how I normally do it today, and then I will try that new thing out tomorrow." Change takes a little bit of work to adapt to in the beginning, but once you get used to it, especially when adopting the use of a new tool, it makes your life easier.

I mentioned a few tools you can use throughout the book already, but I wanted to bring them all together in one chapter so that you have an easy reference to return to, if you want to look back for more information on this later.

In this chapter, we will bring together tools to aid in your journey toward better physical, emotional, and spiritual health.

Keep on Walking

One of the most important things we can do for ourselves is what? I know you know, because I have said it a lot in this book. I also know you know because you have probably heard it a million times in your life already.

If you don't use it, you'll lose it!

Staying physically fit is one of the most important things we can do for ourselves. You have to push yourself to keep moving even if it feels like you can't. It is so easy to succumb to all of the excuses:

1. My body hurts too much today; I will do it tomorrow.

2. If I push myself to do too much, I may hurt myself.

3. I walked yesterday; I do not need to do it today.

4. I am too down to bother. I will start again when I feel better.

5. This is not working; I am just getting worse.

6. I did not work out for most of my life, so why should I start now?

It feels good in the moment to let yourself rest; but in the long run, you will suffer more. It is harder to get yourself in shape when you have let yourself go. The best thing is to keep going. I am not saying you should not listen to your body when it is hurting and asking you for help. What I am saying is to keep active by giving yourself the tools you need to succeed.

Physical Tools to Make Walking Easier

1. Walking Aids

I know it is hard sometimes to admit that you need help. I also know that accepting the use of a walking aid is difficult. There is something about having to use a cane or a walker that feels like you are sliding down a slippery slope. You may feel like you do not want others to see you with it. You may feel like it makes you look weak or old or sick. If you are like 99.999% of people I have met, you will resist using a walking aid in the beginning.

I completely understand. The first time I was told to use a cane while recovering from an injury, I resisted too. I was determined to recover on my own, and I did not want to be dependent on a walking aid for the rest of my life. So, I get it.

The second time I was told to use a cane, I was far less resistant. Why? Because I realized I was so much more confident with it than I was without. I walked more when I was not worrying about my balance. I walked more because I was not afraid of re-injuring myself.

It is important to keep moving, and if you are afraid of moving, then you will not do it. You will use your fear as an excuse to not move at all, and that is the worst possible thing you can do for yourself.

Make It Easy

Some of the limiting beliefs that stop you from accepting a walking aid are:

1. Other people will think I look old.

2. Using a walking aid makes me look sick.

3. If I start using a walking aid, I will have to use one for the rest of my life.

4. Using a walking aid is admitting defeat.

5. Accepting a walking aid is the beginning of the end of my life.

Yes, those are some very heavy thoughts. No wonder a lot of people resist using a cane or a walker. I get it. Like I said, I resisted too. But the thing I want you to ask yourself is: *Do I want to keep walking at all?*

Without the aid, you may fall and injure yourself, making it a whole lot harder to get back on your feet. I ask you this: Would you rather go through the pain of an injury and the subsequent recovery, or would you take the help you need to stay healthy and active?

I really, REALLY hope you chose the latter. If not, maybe the following reframe will help:

1. Using a walker helps me stay active. It does not matter what other people think.

2. Using a walker makes me look smart.

3. If I use a walking aid, I will feel confident in my walking, and therefore do more of it.

4. Using a walking aid is embracing courage, strength, and determination.

5. Accepting a walking aid is the beginning of better health and a higher quality of life.

6. Using a walking aid does not change who I am.

USING A CANE OR A WALKER DOES NOT CHANGE WHO YOU ARE. You are the person who cares enough about themselves to know when you need the help to maintain good health. You have the strength. You have the courage. You have the perseverance. Sometimes using that walking aid will allow you to regain better balance and mobility, meaning that you will not have to use it forever.

2. Pedometer

Another really great tool is one that helps you record and keep track of your progress. A pedometer is a tool you wear that keeps track of the number of steps you take in a day. Most people wear them on their wrist, and the cost can range anywhere from $15 to $300. You really do not need anything fancy to get you started. If you have a smartphone, you can also download an app that will keep track of your steps for you; just remember to keep that phone on you when walking.

Do you have a walking goal? I always think that it is a good thing to set a goal that is measurable in order to track your progress. Let's take the following, really easy example to get you started:

1. Set a goal of walking for 10 minutes. After the first day, record the number of steps you took in those 10 minutes. Set that as your base to hit for the next week. For now, let's say you can hit 50 steps per minute; so in that 10-minute period, you are taking 500 steps.

2. Give yourself a goal to increase the number of steps you take each day by 200 per week. So if you start walking this week, for the entire week, your goal is to hit 500 steps every day. Next week, for the entire week, your goal is to hit 700 steps every single day. For the week after that, your goal is to hit 900 steps every single day. I think you see where I am headed with this.

3. You can increase your number of steps by either increasing the amount of time you walk for or your speed. This is up to your comfort level.

Always remember, when you set your goal, to set a realistic one. The main reason people fail when they begin attempting to achieve a fitness goal is because they set the bar way too high. Be kind to yourself. Start at a reasonable pace, even if it feels too easy, and continue to make it bigger. If you start with a smaller goal and are feeling like you want to do more one day, go for it. You do not have to stop yourself from doing more, but keeping the goal reasonable to start ensures that you will be able to hit that goal.

Mindset Tools to Make Walking Easier

I touched on this idea when addressing the perspective shift that needs to happen when embracing the use of a walking aid. I want to go a little further with this now, looking specifically at walking and how we make it hard on ourselves to succeed.

Just like when you do not accept the help of an aid that will ensure you do not fall, and that will give you the confidence to stay active when your balance is not as good as it used to be, because of how it will make you look or feel about life, you might be letting some limiting beliefs get in your way of walking. I know you want to feel good. I also know that you have the work ethic to succeed. You are letting your limiting beliefs get in the way.

I am going to share with you some of the limiting beliefs that stop people from walking as much as they could:

I am too out of shape to start now. It is too late.

I do not want people to see me huffing and puffing. It is embarrassing.

There is nowhere to walk to in the winter.

Walking is boring.

Walking will not do anything for me; I used to run. It is hard to face how much I cannot do now.

Positive reframe of negative beliefs:

I am strong. I am powerful. I have what it takes to get into shape.

I am an inspiration to others who want to take control of their health.

If I cannot go outside to walk, I can walk in my house.

I can always find a way to make walking interesting.

Walking is the most beneficial exercise for my body.

Take a minute to write down 5 things that stop you from walking:

1. _____

2. _____

3. _____

4. _____

5. _____

Positive reframe of those negative beliefs:

1. _____

2. _____

3. _____

4. _____

5. _____

Amazing! Now that you are ready to remove any and all excuses, and to make walking a regular part of your daily routine, set a goal for yourself, and schedule time each and every day to complete that goal. A big part of shifting your mindset is turning it from that thing you *will* do, into that thing that you *are* doing.

If you are ready to start, put this book down now and go for a walk. I promise I will be here waiting for you the minute you get back!

I want to give you one last tool to help you start walking and keep walking:

MAKE IT INTERESTING!

Get yourself a pair of headphones for your phone. Download your favorite music. Make sure you love the music and that it will inspire you to move. Download a lot of different music so that it does not get too repetitive.

It is also really helpful to have music with a good beat. Your body will naturally want to move to the beat. This creates an energy in your body that will help you catch the momentum to keep on going, especially when you need a push.

Another great way to make walking interesting is to listen to your favorite podcasts. Having something else to focus on helps you stop thinking about some of the negative things you may be feeling, like pain, tiredness, or wishing it was over. You want to help yourself come to a place where you enjoy and even look forward to your daily walks.

Physical Tools for Stretching and Weightlifting

A great way to supplement your daily walking is with stretching and weightlifting. There are many tools you can find online that will help you with either of these.

For stretching, one of the best tools is the resistance band. A resistance band is a latex band that you can get in a range of strengths. You can use this tool to both strengthen your muscles and bring more flexibility back to stiff muscles.

There are a lot of different exercises you can do in the comfort of your own home. You do not even need to commit a long amount of time to them. Some of them you can even do in bed as a part of your morning routine before you get up.

To get exercises, you can either schedule a few sessions with a personal trainer at your local community center, talk to your doctor about meeting with a physical therapist, or watch easy-to-follow YouTube videos, but do not do anything that you do not understand, feels dangerous, or goes against the advice of your doctor.

Weightlifting is something that is also an easy and less time-consuming activity, which you can also do in your own home. I have even incorporated them into my walking, by either buying weights that I could strap onto my feet or carrying weights in my hands.

Follow the same advice as above for learning about the ways you can incorporate weights into your daily exercise routine. A really fun thing that both of these tools can do is help you get creative while moving. Creativity makes everything fun. If you find you are getting bored, and this is making it harder for you to stay motivated to keep active, incorporate any one of these props, and you will find a renewed sense of fun in your workout.

Physical Tools to Make It Easier Around the House

We have spoken about these earlier in the book, but I feel they are important, so I wanted to pull them all together here for you again.

For the bathroom:

If you are struggling with keeping on top of your personal hygiene, it could be because you feel your balance is not as good as it once was, and so you do not shower as often as you should. The best thing to do is to have an occupational therapist come and assess your space to make sure you have the right equipment installed.

Bars on the walls to hold onto as you get in and out from the shower can be very useful in helping you feel more confident. A bar that you can grab onto while you are showering is also good. Another option would be to get a shower bench for the days when you would feel more comfortable sitting while you shower.

Another really helpful tool for the bathroom is to get a raised seat for the toilet. Some toilets are way too short, making it painful to sit, and difficult to get back up. A raised seat alleviates both of these issues.

General tools:

Do you ever find it difficult to pick up things that you have dropped on the floor? There is a handy tool, appropriately named the Reacher Grabber, for getting to those things that are hard to reach. There are many different brands, so it is best to look up the one that suits your needs.

One last, really handy tool is the long shoe horn. This takes away all of the frustration of trying to get on shoes that do not easily just slip right on.

Physical Tools to Keep Your Overall Health on Track

Yes, yes, we just talked a lot about this in the monitoring chapter, so I will not harp on it too much again here. You know you need to monitor both your blood sugar and blood pressure on a daily basis. I recommend getting a container to keep them organized, together with a journal to record your numbers.

The journal is a great tool for you to keep track of your progress. Get one that has sections, or buy divider stickers and organize your book into sections. Keep it simple, and have sections for:

1. Blood sugar

2. Blood pressure

3. Weight

4. Walking steps

5. Big wins!

In that last section, write about your big and small successes. This should be your "feel good" section. On the days when you are feeling like you have not made progress, you can head back to this section and lift your spirits. Be kind to yourself; and always, ALWAYS celebrate your wins.

I also have a separate calendar to schedule the things I am monitoring on different days of the week. I also use this to schedule in my walks, other physical activities, personal hygiene, classes, social engagements, networking events, and rest time.

Creating a schedule of events reminds me of what I need to do. It is also a great way of monitoring my progress. On the days when I do not attend a social event because I am not feeling up to it, I mark it in the calendar. I do not do this to make myself feel bad, but more so that I can look back and see if I have been declining social events for a while. If I am unwilling to admit that I am becoming depressed, this is a really good indicator.

One last tool that can help you keep on track is one that has to do with your medication. If you have multiple medications or supplements to be taken each day, it can be hard to remember if you have taken them. At the beginning of each week, take all of your medications and organize them in a *dosette box*. There are different ones, depending on your needs. For example, you can get one that just has a section for each day of the week, or you can get one that has an AM and PM compartment for each day. Make sure to get the one that makes it easy for you to check and see if you have taken the pills you need to take, at the right time of day.

Inspire Yourself to Eat Well!

The absolute best tool for inspiring yourself to eat well is to give yourself inspiration! How do you give yourself inspiration? I will give you a hint: I have been doing it at the end of each chapter.

You got it! Get yourself some good recipes. Be sure to find cookbooks that are diabetic friendly. There are even books that are written specifically to address your needs. New and exciting recipes make eating healthy way more fun.

Help yourself enjoy eating again. Food brings joy. It's all about making it fun, and savoring the flavors. Let those who love food, inspire you to get creative in the kitchen.

Emotional Tools for Overall Success

We have talked about looking to your family, friends, and network for support. We have also talked about the importance of being kind to yourself. One last tool I want to share with you in this chapter is one that has helped millions to change their habits. Thought patterns, built over long periods of time, strengthen and become difficult to change.

If you are used to reaching for a can of sugary soda at 3pm to get you through the afternoon slump, it will be hard to break that habit. Something that can help you is affirmations and mindset work. There are many mindset leaders who are experts in the field. I want to give you a small taste of it here, and then you can decide if you want to seek out more resources in the field.

I believe that two of the most important things you can do as you are making the change to lead a healthier life, are:

1. Love yourself unconditionally.
2. Raise your confidence in yourself.

To begin your mindset work, I want you to answer these questions:

1. How do I show myself that I love myself every single day?

2. What actions does the confident version of me take every day?

Answer these questions in the present tense. Answer them as many times as you like.

Answers for question 1:

- I show myself that I love myself by speaking kindly to myself.

- I show myself that I love myself by celebrating my wins.

- I show myself that I love myself by wearing clothes that make me feel great.

- I show myself that I love myself by honoring my boundaries.

Answers for question 2:

- My confidence allows me to take a new class.

- My confidence allows me to join a walking group.

- My confidence allows me to take a break when I need to.

Once you are done answering each question as many times as you can, either write out or say the following affirmations out loud:

My life is worth it.
I am an amazing human being.
I deserve to have all that I desire in life.
I know that I always make the right decisions.
I am loved and freely share my love.

Spiritual Tools for Overall Success

For me, it is very important to connect with God. I am grateful for my life, and I engage in that practice every single day. To help myself stay active in this practice, I use a prayer book. It gives me a prayer for every single day, and pairs it with the reading of a scripture. This practice lifts my mood and reminds me that I am not alone. I have a purpose, and I am being watched over.

It does not matter what you believe in; you can develop a practice like this for yourself too. One thing you can do every day is think about what you are grateful for in your life. Again, you can either write it out or say it out loud. You can think about as many things as you like; in fact, the more the better. The longer you live in gratitude each day, the easier it is to recognize the positives in your life.

You are here for a purpose.
Your life is important.
You matter!

Give Yourself the Tools!

You are here because you want to succeed. You have made it to the end of this book because you are ready to do the work. You are inspired to take your health back and kick diabetes in the behind, so arm yourself with the tools you need in order to ensure your success. Take care of yourself physically, mentally, and spiritually!

Health-Happy Celebration Meal

Since this is a celebration, I have included a few of my favorite recipes for you!

RECIPE #1

Butternut Squash with Cumin Couscous

Ingredients

1 butternut squash (about 2 pounds)
2 tablespoons olive oil
1 large yellow onion, diced
2 cloves garlic, finely chopped
1/4 teaspoon cayenne pepper
1/8 teaspoon ground cinnamon

1/8 teaspoon ground nutmeg
1 teaspoon cumin
1 cup canned diced tomatoes
1/3 cup dark or golden raisins
1 32-ounce container of vegetable broth (water)
1 15.5-ounce can chickpeas, rinsed and drained
2 teaspoons kosher salt
1 1/2 cups couscous
2 tablespoons fresh chopped flat-leaf parsley leaves
1/4 cup almonds, chopped

How to Make

Half and peel the squash. Remove seeds and cut the squash into 1-inch chunks. Heat the oil in a Dutch oven or saucepan, over medium heat. Add the onion and cook for 5 minutes. Add the garlic, cayenne, cinnamon, nutmeg, and 1/2 teaspoon cumin, and cook for 1 minute. Stir in the squash, tomatoes, raisins, broth or water, chickpeas, and 1 1/2 teaspoons of the salt. Bring to a boil. Reduce heat, cover, and simmer for 10 minutes. Uncover and cook until the squash is tender (15–20 minutes).

Meanwhile, in a medium saucepan, bring 1 1/2 cups of water to a boil, adding the remaining cumin and salt. Stir in the couscous. Cover, remove from heat, and let stand for 5–10 minutes. Fluff with a fork.

To service: Dish couscous into a bowl and top with squash. Sprinkle with parsley and almonds.

RECIPE #2

Chayote Salad
AKA Cho Cho Salad

Ingredients

2 chayote / cho cho
Vinaigrette Dressing:
1 tablespoon champagne vinegar or
        white vinegar or
        rice vinegar
3 tablespoons olive oil
1 shallot, finely chopped
1 large clove of garlic, crushed and finely chopped
2 scallions, sliced thin
1/2 teaspoon pineapple juice
1/8 teaspoon hot sauce
Season with salt and pepper.

Method:

Cut the chayote / cho cho in half [lengthwise]. Remove the core, and with a knife, peel the skin. Cut chayote/cho cho into cubes.

Cook the chayote / cho cho cubes in salted water for 10–15 minutes. Do not overcook. Make sure the chayote/cho cho cubes are still crunchy.

While the chayote / cho cho is cooking, prepare the dressing by mixing the vinegar, oil, shallot, garlic, scallions, pineapple juice, hot sauce, and salt and pepper.

Remove the chayote / cho cho cubes and drain well. Place in a bowl and toss with dressing.

Serve immediately.

RECIPE #3

Curry Goat

Ingredients

2 kg goat stew meat, cut into 2.5cm/1-inch pieces
3 tbsp. curry powder
1 tbsp. cooking oil
1 tbsp. curry powder for burning
½ tsp. cumin (optional)
1 tsp. fennel seeds (optional)
1 tbsp. salt, leveled or to taste
½ tsp. black pepper
½ tsp. allspice, ground
1 tbsp. onion powder, unsalted
1 tbsp. garlic powder, unsalted
½ tbsp. soya sauce, MSG-free
1 tbsp. Worcestershire sauce, MSG-free (optional)
1-inch-thick ginger root or 1 teaspoon ginger powder
½ medium scotch bonnet pepper
1 large onion, chopped

6 cloves garlic, crushed
½ large bell pepper, diced
1 bunch thyme
6 stalks scallion, chopped
6–8 pimento seeds
1 medium Irish potato, diced

Instructions

In a large bowl, rinse the goat stew meat in vinegar or lime or lemon juice, and then drain completely.

Season the goat stew meat with salt, black pepper, curry powder, allspice, onion powder, garlic powder, ginger powder, soya sauce, and Worcestershire sauce.

Prep (cut) fresh herbs and spices (onion, garlic, thyme, bell pepper, scallion, etc.), and add half the portion to the goat stew meat.

Thoroughly rub all the seasoning into the goat stew meat, by hand or by using a large utensil.

Cover and let marinate for 6–8 hours, or move immediately to the next step.

In a large skillet, heat cooking oil on medium heat.

Immediately add 1 tablespoon of the curry powder, and stir quickly and thoroughly for approximately 15 seconds.

Add the seasoned goat stew meat, stir for 30 seconds, cover the pot, and let cook for 3 minutes.

Next, add enough boiling water to cover the goat stew meat. Cover the pot and cook on high heat for 2 ½ to 3 hours.

Remember to check and stir the pot every 10 minutes, ensuring the water does not dry out too much.

Each time your water runs low, add more boiling water to completely cover the goat stew meat until the meat is cooked.

After approximately 2 ¾ hours, test a small piece of the goat stew meat to see if it has the desired texture and saltiness. Add more salt (to taste) if needed.

When your goat meat is completely soft/cooked, add the Irish potatoes, the second portion of chopped seasoning, and 1 cup boiling water. Cover and cook on medium-high heat for a further 8–10 minutes.

When your potatoes are tender, reduce heat to medium, stir the pot, and then leave it uncovered to allow the gravy to thicken (approximately 5 minutes).

When the gravy has the desired consistency, re-cover the pot (for 3–5 minutes) and let the curry goat absorb all the delicious flavors from the gravy!

Serve hot, bless up, and enjoy it!

RECIPE #4

Raw Beetroot and Carrot Salad Recipe

1 large/medium raw beetroot {grated}
2 medium carrots {grated}
2 tbsp. {handful} of sultana raisins
1 tbsp. sesame seeds
1 tbsp. sunflower seeds
1 tbsp. extra virgin olive oil
1/4 tsp. cumin
Salt and pepper to taste
Mix all ingredients in a bowl, and sprinkle with sunflower seeds to serve.

RECIPE #5

Brown Rice and Swiss Chard

2 tablespoons butter or oil
1/2 red onion, chopped
1–2 tablespoons water
1 1/2 cups cooked brown rice
1 large bunch Swiss chard, stalk removed, chopped
{or about 5–6 large and 3–4 small leaves}
1/4 teaspoon salt
1 tablespoon soy sauce
2 teaspoons balsamic vinegar

Sauté first 3 ingredients in a large pan until the onion is tender, about 5 minutes.

Add rice, and then carefully add water so that it doesn't spit all over you. Place chard on top; cover to let chard steam, for about 5 minutes or until chard is tender.

If you are using spinach, do not add the water. Just place chopped spinach on top of rice, and cover for 1–2 minutes or until spinach wilts.

Add soy sauce and vinegar, and stir thoroughly.

Enjoy!!!!

RECIPE #6

Carrot Cake

Ingredients

1 cup salad oil
1/4 cup butter
2 cups brown sugar
4 eggs
2 cups sifted flour
2 tsp. baking powder
2 tsp. baking soda
2 tsp. cinnamon
1/4 tsp. nutmeg
1/2 tsp. salt
1 tsp. vanilla
1 cup chopped pecans or walnuts (optional)

2 cups grated carrots
1 cup shredded carrots
1/2 cup shredded coconut (optional)
1/2 cup cranberries
1 cup raisins

Directions

Blend oil, butter, and sugar until fluffy. Add eggs one at a time. Mix all dry ingredients and add to the mixture. Blend well. Add remaining ingredients. Pour into 3, 9-inch greased and floured cake pans. Or you could choose to bake it all in one large pan. Bake at 350°F for 25 minutes or until done.

CHAPTER 10

The 11-Step Program

*Because You Deserve
Better Health*

"I believe that the greatest gift that you can give your family and the world is a healthy you."

– Joyce Meyer

10

Your health is your greatest wealth! Without a doubt, I believe that the best thing you can do for yourself and the world around you is to take care of your health. When you feel great, you can do great things.

I do not know about you, but I want to do great things, and this is one of the reasons why health is so important to me. But not only that, I want to wake up every day feeling the best I can possibly feel. I want to do this for myself. I want you to do it for yourself. When you take your health seriously, you ultimately lead by example.

The better you treat yourself, the better others will treat you.

The better you treat yourself, the better others will treat themselves.

You are in control of your health, and if anyone has the power to achieve better health, it is you. You have taken the time to read through this whole book. How are you doing with implementing what I have talked about? I do not say learned, because I believe deep down that you already know a lot about what your body, mind, and soul need to feel great each day. That said, sometimes we all need a little outside inspiration to remind us that we have many options. Often, we need a reminder that we do not have to go it alone. I hope that this book serves as that reminder for you.

Good Health Is a Priority

Throughout my life, I have always recognized the importance of taking care of myself. This is not to say that there have not been times when I have struggled. I am not perfect. But in the end, I have taken the time to figure out what I need to do to get me back on track, and have put in the effort to do it.

WHY?

1. Because I love myself.

2. Because I value my life.

3. Because I want to give myself the opportunity to live my very best life.

4. Because I love my family.

5. Because I know I have a lot to offer the world.

6. Because I want to lead by example.

WHY SHOULD YOU MAKE YOUR HEALTH A PRIORITY?

1. Because you love yourself.

2. Because you value your life.

3. Because you want to give yourself the opportunity to live your very best life.

4. _____

5. _____

Yes, I have left spaces where you can fill in the rest. You are the most important person in your world, so you have to be the one to put your health first. It is a simple choice. It is one your life depends on.

It is never too late. What I can do is share with you a lifetime of experience in establishing and maintaining healthy habits. As you have seen in this book, I have a wealth of experience and knowledge. It all comes from personal experience and growth. But not only that, it is also dedication and passion. I am passionate about my health. I am dedicated to be in the best possible health I can be. For these reasons, both family and friends have always come to me when they need some help.

My sister's journey to better health, after a diabetes diagnosis, inspired me to continue to learn more about the ways in which I could reach out beyond my circle and use my knowledge to help others as well. This is where the inspiration for this book came from. I want as many people as possible in this world to know that achieving better health does not have to be hard; all you have to do is set yourself up for success.

Good Health Takes Just as Much Effort as Bad Health

When you think about it, does it feel easier or harder to maintain a healthy lifestyle? At first thought, you might think it is easier to maintain the unhealthy one. It is easy to grab a bottle of pop in the mid-afternoon to get you through low energy. It is easy to drive through and pick up some fast food on the way home. It is easy to sit on the couch and turn on the TV. Yes, you're right. At this moment, those choices feel easier, because they are habits. You are used to them. You have been doing them every day for years now.

I argue that living a healthy lifestyle is not hard at all, once you get in the habit of it. It is the transition that feels like work; but once you are there, it is easy. There is nothing tastier than fresh fruit in the morning. I promise that once you get used to your new lifestyle, you will understand what you have been missing out on.

I would even go so far as to argue that you will realize that your unhealthy lifestyle choices actually made your life much harder. Think about that afternoon sugar fix. How long did you actually feel good for after it? With every quick *sugar high*, comes an even lower *sugar low*. If you feel tired in the afternoon, and the option is available to you, it would be better for you to take a quick 10-minute nap. Don't stay longer though! Just take a quick 10 minutes to rest, even if you don't sleep, and then you should feel better than you did, for much longer than if you had put a bunch of sugar in your body.

You have begun the work by reading this book, and maybe you have even made some great progress in changing your daily routines, but now comes the hard part. Now comes the part where you are done reading this book, and you have to stick to the 11 steps on your own. What do you need to set yourself up with to succeed?

Let us take a moment to review the 11 steps, and see where you are at. Do you need support? What kind of support do you need?

11 Steps to Achieving Better Health

1. **Understand the foods that are good for your body.**

   Sometimes we make poor health choices because we really do not know what is best for us. Generally, we understand that processed foods, like fast foods, are terrible for our health, and that eating a large amount of sugary treats is not good either, but understanding what is truly good for your body may take a little bit of trial and error. This is the perfect time to try out new and interesting foods. Find healthy options that you really love. The main takeaway I have for you is: Listen to your body. It is speaking to you. It is telling you what it needs.

2. **Remove the unhealthy food choices from your diet.**

   This will be one of the biggest lifestyle changes you make for your health. It is all about mindset. You are determined to change your health for the better. You are ready to face the challenges. You are ready to take control of your life. The right mindset is one that reflects all of these things you are ready for. Your actions will then be based on that mindset. It is not only a strong mindset you need; you have to set yourself up for success by removing all of the temptations from your home.

3. **Learn how to prepare fresh food in your home.**

   The best way to avoid fast foods is to learn how to make food that you like. Shift your mindset from, "I am hungry; what can I find to satisfy that hunger right now?" to "What delicious food can I begin preparing for when I am hungry later today?" Have good, healthy options in your home. You do not have to become a master chef. All of the menus I have shared in this book are easy to prepare and take very little time. Once you get in the habit of making your own food, you will realize how satisfying it is, even if you do not have a burning desire to cook all of the time.

4. **Stay active. If you do not use it, you will lose it!**

That said, it is never too late to start. Be kind to yourself throughout the process. Reward yourself, in a healthy way, for all that you do. Start slow and work your way up. The most important thing to do is to choose activities you love. Find fun ways to get yourself inspired, like watching a YouTube video to dance in your living room, or listening to an interesting podcast while you go for a walk. There are so many fun ways to get your body moving, and the more you do it, the easier it will become.

5. **Take care of your personal hygiene.**

When you look good, you feel good. When you feel good, you participate in life in a more active way. Wear clothes you feel great in and are clean. Dress up once in a while. Enjoy the way you feel. Taking care of yourself is the most important step in beginning your self-love journey. Spend the time to make yourself feel great!

6. **Establish a positive mindset.**

    This does not mean that you have to shove all your negative feelings deep inside and never ever express them or recognize them. What it does mean is that you understand them and work on releasing them so that you can step into the amazing aspects of your life. You are already helping yourself become more positive by taking control of your eating habits, getting active, and taking care of your personal hygiene. Living your life in a positive frame of mind will then in turn help you be even more successful in achieving your health and fitness goals.

7. **Make your mental health a priority.**

    Achieving better mental health is about so much more than mindset. Depression is a real concern, especially when you are worried about your health. Going through major shifts in lifestyle choices can at first seem overwhelming, but once you get going, it does get easier. Throughout the process, stay aware of your moods. If you are feeling so low that it is difficult to get out of bed, do not beat yourself up. Get help!

8. **Incorporate social activities into your life.**

    Humans are social beings. Yes, some of us are more social than others, but it is important to push yourself to get out and see people once in a while. It is a win-win for everyone. Your day is made better by having been with others, and their day is made better by having been with you. Also, having events to look forward to is great for your mental health. Events can break up the monotony of your daily routine. They give you something to look forward to. Look for new events to attend, where you will meet new people. Whatever you do, stay social!

9. **Monitor your health daily.**

   Slipping back into old patterns can be a slow and almost unnoticeable process at first, and then suddenly it hits you; you have slid down the slippery slope, and now you have so much work to do to get back to where you were. Similarly, depression does not just turn up in a day; it can creep up on you slowly, until one day you cannot get out of bed. Monitoring is a great tool to keep on top of all your health needs: physical, mental, emotional, and spiritual.

10. **Get the tools you need to achieve optimal physical, spiritual, and mental health.**

    Make this journey to better health easy on yourself. There are so many tools you can give yourself to make this transition easier. I know I say this a lot, but set yourself up for success, every single day. It does not have to be hard. You have the power to make it easy, and maybe even a lot of fun. The tools will help you stay on track and reach your goals. Some tools are physical tools, like walking aids to allow you to stay confident in your balance, and to keep you active. Other tools can be a recipe book to help you stay creative in the kitchen, or spiritual readings to help you stay connected to your faith.

11. **Get the support you need to succeed.**

You do not have to do this alone. There is so much help available to you. It is up to you to ask for the help you need. Start with family and then friends. If you do not find all that you need, reach out to the community. Join a support group or a social group. See a therapist or hire a coach. If you truly want to reach your goal, you need help. There is no need to go it alone! Surround yourself with a support network that will be there for you no matter what.

Get the Support You Need

I am here for you! If you have found this book helpful, and you know that you need some ongoing support to keep you on the path you have begun with me here,

I have a few offerings to provide you with continued support as you navigate this journey further.

I offer 1:1 coaching support, either over Zoom if you are in another part of the world, or in-person support if you are located near me. Both options are effective! I work with you to become even stronger in your work on each of the 11 steps. That said, I customize my program to suit you. If you need more help or encouragement to eat healthier than you do, or to stay on top of your personal hygiene, we will focus more on that. You are the driver. I am here to keep you on route to a healthier version of you.

Here are a few things I do to specifically help my clients achieve success with the 11 Steps to Achieve Better Health program:

1. Assess eating habits at the outset of our work together, and come up with a new plan.

2. Provide recipe suggestions and resources.

3. Be available for encouragement and support throughout the process.

4. Encourage you to find new social events in your area or online.

5. Help you monitor your physical, mental, and spiritual health.

6. Work with you to come up with a realistic and fun exercise schedule.

7. Listen when you need to talk.

I am here for you. If you want to find out more about my service, you can find out more information on my website: **wellnesscoachbook.com.** If you would like to speak to me about your needs, I would love to chat. Send me an e-mail, at **pauline@wellnesscoachbook.com,** and I will get back to you as soon as I can.

Why I Do What I Do

> *"Each time a person passes by you and you say 'hello,' imagine that person turning into a candle. The more positivity, love, and light you reflect, the more light is mirrored your way. Sharing beautiful hellos is the quickest way to earn spiritual brownie points. You should start seeing hellos as small declarations of faith. Every time you say hello to a stranger, your heart acknowledges over and over again that we are all family."*
>
> **– Suzy Kassem**

I love people. I love helping people. It is my legacy in this life to be the person who lifts others up and provides them with the support they need to achieve their health goals.

It is my belief that we are all here for a purpose. You have a purpose in this world. You are important. Your life matters. When you do not allow yourself the opportunity to realize that purpose, the world is missing out. When you do not take care of yourself, you are not able to live your purpose to the fullest, and this is when the world misses out.

The world misses out on all of the amazing things you have to offer just by being you. When you are living each day in optimal health, you are allowing your light to shine. You are a living example for others.

I am the person who is here to help all those who want to bring themselves back to better health, so that they too can live their legacy and make this world an even better place to live. The more I am able to live my purpose, the more others are able to live their purpose, and the movement spreads. The goodness grows and expands out beyond your immediate network.

Love, health, and happiness are powerful creators of positive energy. When you are healthy, you help to create that energy. I am here to help you come back to a place where you can do that. I have faith in you.

How did I know this was my calling? I did not at first. I just loved helping people because I knew that I could. I have built a lifetime of knowledge on healthy living. I have always been excited and happy to share that knowledge with others. Because I was passionate about it, I would talk about it, but I did not think to make it my mission to share my knowledge with the world. I just did what I did because I liked doing it.

When people started coming to me with their health questions, at first I was really surprised. I did not understand why they thought I would have the answer. I soon began to understand what was happening. Most often, I did have the answer, and I loved spending the time to share my knowledge with anyone who needed it. If I did not know the answer, I would find it. I never wanted to leave anyone needing help and not receiving the help they needed. If I could not provide them with what they needed, then I would find someone who could.

I LOVE what I do, because I think that if everyone on this planet could feel the difference a healthy lifestyle makes, they would not hesitate to do it. Living in an unhealthy body is so much harder, every single day, than the work you will have to put in to change your habits. You have the strength, the courage, and the determination. I believe that you and everyone in this world can change their habits to live healthier. In the long run, you will be so grateful you did.

Can you imagine waking up every day with more energy?

Can you imagine what it would feel like to know you gave yourself the opportunity to be your very best every day?

Can you imagine all that you could accomplish in this world if you stopped getting in your own way?

You would be unstoppable. I believe in the power within you. This is why I do what I do! I love people, and I love seeing them thrive. This is my passion and my purpose: To see as many people as I possibly can, thriving in their lives because they have taken control of their health.

Is this you? Are you ready to take control of your life? Are you ready to implement the 11 steps to achieve better health? Do you know you need some support?

I am here for you!

You Are Your #1 Priority

One of the biggest lessons you will need to learn, if you have not already, is how to put yourself first. People hold onto a whole range of limiting beliefs that have taught them it is selfish, bad, or greedy to put your needs before others. I am here to tell you that those beliefs are not only limiting; they are 100% wrong.

You are meant to put yourself first. It is where you begin; it is your baseline—it is your starting place! When you put your need for greater health above all else, you will begin to make the choices you need to make in order to achieve your goals. When you achieve these goals, you then can be there more for the people you love. But first, you have to think of you.

I do not normally write out affirmations, but if you are struggling to put your health above all else that you do, having a few mantras to repeat throughout the day might help to remind you why you are putting the effort in now to live a healthier life.

Here are a few simple but effective affirmations:

1. I am important.

2. I matter.

3. My life is important.

4. I value my health.

5. I get to decide the outcome.

6. Today is my day to thrive.

7. I live with purpose.

8. The universe is always looking out for me.

9. I am unique.

10. I provide value to this world.

11. I am here for a reason.

When you read these, how do they make you feel? Do you believe it when you read it, say it, or write it? If you find your brain proving these affirmations wrong, you may want to do some more inner work. Take some time and ask yourself these questions:

1. What is my most amazing accomplishment?

2. Why am I proud of this accomplishment?

3. What is one memory of a time when the universe provided what I needed in the moment?

4. What is one unique quality I possess? Remember that this quality is unique to you, even if others possess it. For example, if you can carry a show tune in the shower, no-one else can do it like you.

These are just a few ideas to get you started. In all honesty, understanding your worth and putting your life first is a topic that could take a whole book or two to cover. If you feel you need to work on this more, you know what to do: ASK FOR HELP!

The bottom line is that you need to put yourself first in order to make your health a top priority!

Welcome to a happier, healthier you!

Now that you are ready to put yourself first, even if you need to work on it, and you have some tools to get you started, you are on the path to achieving better health. It is time to celebrate. You might want to treat yourself to one of the meals I shared with you in the last chapter. Or put on your dancing shoes and go out for a fun night with friends. Whatever you choose to do, I hope you truly give yourself the credit you deserve for embarking on this journey.

Remember that if you need any help or would like to share your wins with me, I would love to hear from you **(wellnesscoachbook.com)**.

Before I go, I would like to leave you with two bonus recipes. I have saved the very best for last, so make sure you give these a try!

Dona's Diabetic Shot

Ingredients:

1 cup ginger juice
1 cup shredded garlic juice
1 cup apple cider vinegar
1 cup lemon juice
3 tablespoons honey {preferably raw}

Method:

In a blender, blend lemon juice with garlic, and pour into a saucepan.

Blend ginger with apple cider vinegar, and pour into a saucepan.

Boil mixture over medium heat for half an hour. Sweeten with honey.

Cool and pour into glass bottles/jars, and place in the refrigerator.

Adjust liquidity by adding more lemon juice and apple cider vinegar if necessary.

Also, adjust sweetness {not too sweet}.

Take 1 tablespoon every morning before breakfast.

Note:

If you do not own a juicer, for the ginger juice, you can blend 1 and a half cups of shredded ginger with the apple cider vinegar. Apply above procedure and strain through double cheesecloth or a clean white tea towel. Thoroughly squeeze all the juice.

Enjoy!!!!

Immune Buster Shot

1 cup chopped, washed, skin-on ginger

1 cup chopped, washed, skin-on turmeric

1/2 cup apple cider vinegar

1 medium onion

1 lemon with most of the peel on {not too much of the peel, and remove lemon seeds}

3 large cloves of garlic

Dash of cayenne pepper

2 tablespoons honey, or to taste

Method:

Combine all ingredients in a blender or a bullet, and blend until liquefied.

Do not add water.

Strain through a clean white tea towel. Squeeze out all of the juice into a glass jar.

Place in the refrigerator.

Take 1 shot glass in the morning and one in the evening.

When taken on an empty stomach, you can feel the warmth all through your stomach.

ACKNOWLEDGMENTS

Thank you to my children: **Kwabena El, Steve Bryan, Rosette Bryan, and Kirk Bryan.** You are always there for me when I need you, giving me the encouragement I need to dream big and go for those dreams. Your love fills me with joy, and inspires me every day to be the best person I can be. I love you all to the moon and back!

Without you, **Amit Ambegaonkar**, this book would not be possible. Thank you for being the kind of mentor who pushes me to take action on my goals. You are a great inspiration, and for that, I am incredibly grateful.

Thank you, **Jessica Chan**, for standing by me when I need you. You are so much more than a mortgage broker to me. I appreciate all of the support you so generously give me.

Christina Fife, thank you for always being there when I had a question or needed to get something done. You are always available to help when you are needed. I appreciate you and all of the work you have done for me. Thank you also, **Liz Ventrella**, for guiding me through this process. You were always patient with me and made everything run so smoothly.

To my amazing, funny, and supportive friends: {**Bibi**} **Joy Khan, Lovina Cummings, and Joan Lee.** Where would we be without each other? You make me laugh. You offer a shoulder when I need it. You encourage me to do the things I want to do. Thanks for being my confidants. Thank you for being my partners in crime. Thank you for being the wonderful people that you are. I am grateful for you!

www.ingramcontent.com/pod-product-compliance
Lightning Source LLC
Chambersburg PA
CBHW062219270326
41930CB00009B/1788